COLOR ATLAS OF HUMAN ORAL HISTOLOGY

Hironori Kitamura, D.D.S., D.Med.Sc., Ph.D.
Professor Emeritus of Oral Histology
Kanagawa Dental College, Yokosuka, Japan

Masatoyo Oda, D.D.S., D.Med.Sc.
Professor of Oral Anatomy
Osaka Dental University, Osaka, Japan

John A. Hess, D.D.S., M.Phil.
Professor of Anatomy
University of Detroit Mercy School of Dentistry
Detroit, Michigan

CONTRIBUTORS

Shigeo Aiyama, Ph.D.
Yoshikage Higashi, D.D.S., D.Med.Sc.
Masatake Imai, D.D.S., D.Med.Sc.
Yoshimi Terake, M.D.
Yoshihisa Toda, D.D.S., D.Med.Sc.

Ishiyaku EuroAmerica, Inc., Publishers
St. Louis · Tokyo

Book Editor: Gregory Hacke, D.C.

Ishiyaku EuroAmerica, Inc.
716 Hanley Industrial Court, St. Louis, Missouri 63144

PHONE ORDERS CALL TOLL FREE 800-MED-1921

Library of Congress Catalogue Number 91-055254

Hironori Kitamura/Masatoyo Oda/John Hess
COLOR ATLAS OF HUMAN ORAL HISTOLOGY

ISBN 0-912791-80-2

Ishiyaku EuroAmerica, Inc.
St. Louis • Tokyo

Composition by: HiTec Typeset, 101 Orr, Columbia, Missouri 65201
Printed in Portugal by: GRÁFICA EUROPAM, LDA

PREFACE

I recently had the opportunity to review the Japanese edition of Kitamura's COLOR ATLAS OF HUMAN ORAL HISTOLOGY. I was particularly excited to examine this atlas since I had felt for a long time that such a text should be available to dental students and others interested in the field of oral histology. The quality of the illustrations and coverage of the material, both of facial embryology and of the oral structures was very impressive. I was delighted to learn that an English-language edition was being considered for publication. It is a privilege to serve as the editor of this English-language edition of the COLOR ATLAS OF HUMAN ORAL HISTOLOGY.

The original Japanese first edition of this Atlas, edited by the late S. Nagahama, was published in 1970. A revised fourth edition, edited by H. Kitamura and M. Oda, was published in 1988 and is the basis of this American edition. The Japanese text was translated into English by Hironori Kitamura, Professor Emeritus of Oral Histology and Embryology at the Dental College of Kanagawa.

Oral histology and facial embryology provides an important basis for all disciplines of clinical dentistry. This atlas will aid in understanding the concepts of growth and development of the face and oral structures.

This atlas is designed for use in the microscopic laboratory to assist the student in the visual identification and differentiation of normal human tissue and in the interpretation of changes that occur during the development of the facial and oral structures. It consists of high quality macroscopic and microscopic photographs of human embryologic structures and mature oral tissues. Each chapter begins with a brief discussion of the material and may include drawings for additional clarification. Each illustration within a chapter is labeled and provided with a legend. Routine hematoxylin and eosin stains of tissues are used in most instances, however, special stains are utilized to illustrate specific features of the tissues. Transmission and scanning electron micrographs are included to provide a greater understanding of cells, tissues and mineralized structures of special significance.

Dr. Kitamura and his group are to be commended on the preparation of the specimens and the superb photomicrographs. This atlas would not be possible without their excellent contributions. In order to maintain a reasonable price, it was necessary to use the original Japanese illustration plates with the English text replacing the Japanese. The text was rewritten to agree with concepts and terminology widely used in the United States.

I wish to express my gratitude to Mr. Manuel Ponte, President of Ishiyaku EuroAmerica, Inc. for his efforts and for sending the Japanese-edition for my examination.

John A. Hess, D.D.S., M.Phil.

PREFACE

A Japanese first edition of the *Color Atlas of Human Oral Histology* was prepared by eight workers, including the late S. Nagahama and myself. It was a collection of color microphotos designed for use in the microscopic laboratory to assist the dental students. Ever since, we have continued to add photos of better quality from new specimens wherever we could. We have also added scanning electron micrographs at every opportunity.

In a revised fourth edition, we presented a number of photos of frontal or sagittal sections obtained fromt the fetal jaws containing tooth buds and a number of illustrations indicating reconstruction models. Preparation procedures, staining procedures and magnification ratio or the scale of enlargement were also rewritten. Further, some legends were added to the microphotos in various places in each chapter.

In the English-language edition, a few microphotos were replaced with better ones and parts of the text were revised. The labeling of various microphotos was changed to a more uniform style.

We wish to thank Dr. J. A. Hess for his assistance in editing this English edition and for his suggestions for improvement.

Hironori Kitamura, D.D.S., D.Med.Sc., Ph.D.

NOTICE

Dentistry is an ever-changing science. As new research and clinical experience broaden our knowledge, changes in treatment are required. The editors and the publisher of this work have made every effort to ensure that the procedures herein are accurate and in accord with the standards accepted at the time of publication.

CONTENTS

1

Development of the Oral Cavity and Teeth

Formation of the Oral Cavity

The formation of the structures of the head and neck requires a complicated migration and interaction of embryonic tissues. These tissues include ectoderm, mesoderm, endoderm, and mesenchyme derived from the cells of the neural crest or ectomesenchyme. For the purpose of clarity, development is described in weeks after fertilization.

During the third week, the prochordal plate or oropharyngeal membrane is overgrown by the rapid expansion of the neural cavity. This proliferation, combined with the external appearance of multiple branchial or pharyngeal arches on the lateral side of the head, creates the center of the developing face, the stomodeum or primitive oral cavity.

By the beginning of the fourth week, the oropharyngeal membrane has ruptured resulting in the communication of the amniotic cavity with the primitive gut. The primordium of the adenohypophysis appears as a midline outpocketing of the oral epithelium called Rathke's pouch. This invagination of epithelium meets a similar extension from the floor of the diencephalon which will form the neurohypophysis (Fig. 1-A: c). On the lateral surface of the frontal eminence, two small circular elevations called nasal placodes becomes evident.

By the fifth week, the oral cavity is surrounded by the frontal eminence and the maxillary and mandibular processes of the first branchial arch (Fig. 1-A; Figs. 1-1-1, 2). At this time, the nasal placodes have become surrounded by the medial and lateral nasal swellings or processes. The resulting depression of the nasal placodes creates the nasal pits. As the nasal pits deepen into sacs, they remain separated from the primitive oral cavity by the oronasal membrane. At the beginning of the sixth week, this membrane ruptures (Figs. 1-3-1, 2). The external openings of the nasal sacs are now called anterior nares and the internal passageways into the primitive mouth cavity are termed the primitive choanae or primary posterior nares. The nasal sacs are now called the primary nasal cavities (Fig. 1-B). During this period, the two medial nasal processes move towards the midline where they fuse to form the intermaxillary segment or the globular process. As these two processes fuse, a horizontal shelf extends posteriorly from the midline. This projection forms the primary palate.

During the middle of the sixth week, the maxillary process expands into the oral cavity as two lateral palatine shelves or processes (Fig. 1-A, Fig. 1-2-2). They are, at first, oriented vertically, one on each side of the developing tongue. With the repositioning of the tongue at the beginning of the seventh week, these shelves assume a horizontal position and grow medially (Fig. 1-6-1, 2). Beginning anteriorly, they fuse with each other and the primary palate. Fusion of the two palatine processes proceeds posteriorly in the midline (Figs. 1-7-1, 2; Fig. 1-C). This union forms the secondary palate which is completed by the end of the eighth week with the formation of the soft palate (Fig. 1-C, Fig. 1-8-1). During this time, fusion also takes place between the newly formed palate and the nasal septum, which is formed by the frontal prominence.

The formation of the secondary palate establishes the secondary nasal cavity or chamber and the definitive oral cavity. The secondary nasal cavities communicate with the primitive pharynx by way of the secondary choanae or the secondary posterior nares.

In the thirteenth week, the rostral ends of the fused epithelial wall of the primary palate and secondary palate form the transitory nasopalatine ducts (Figs. 1-9-1, 2; Fig. 1-D). These structures retrogress before birth (Fig. 1-12-1, Fig. 10-2-1, Fig. 12-3-2). The incisive canal may be considered the midline landmark between the primary and secondary palates.

At about 37 days, another transitory structure, Chievitz's organ, appears near the corner of the mouth (Figs. 1-4-1, 2). It is positioned near the future location of the deciduous second molar tooth germ. About 4 days later, the primordium of the parotid gland is seen as an epithelial ingrowth or bud near the corners of the mouth (Fig. 1-6-1).

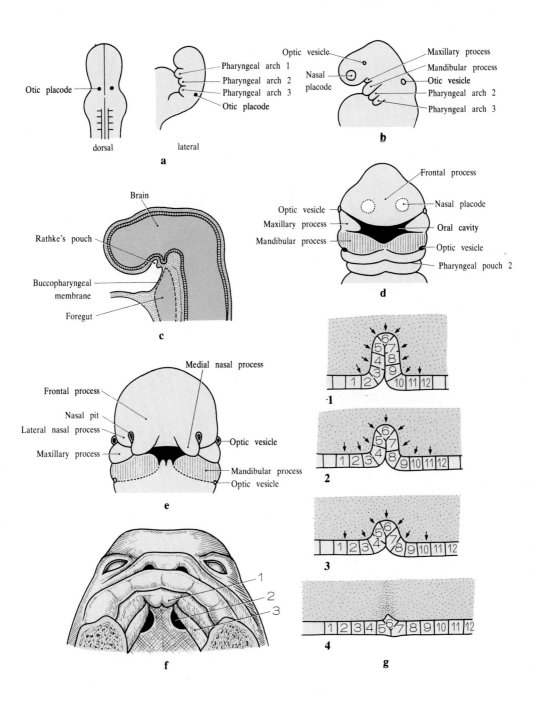

Fig. 1-A Development of the Oral-Facial Complex
a. 20-day human embryo (2mm GL) **b.** 28-day human embryo (4mm GL), lateral view **c.** 26-day human embryo (3.5mm GL), sagittal view **d.** 28-day human embryo (4mm GL), frontal view **e.** 32-day embryo (8mm CR length) **f.** 35-day embryo (13mm CR length) **1.** Primary palate from the globular process **2.** Primary posterior nares **3.** Lateral palatine process **g.** Merging of the maxillary and medial nasal process epithelium.

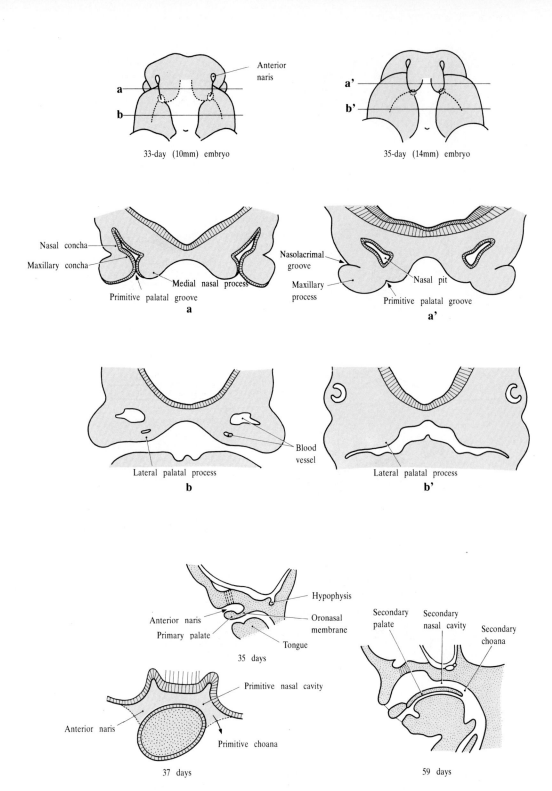

Fig. 1-B The development of the nasal cavity and palate are illustrated in this sagittal section of the head. At 37 days the oronasal membrane ruptures forming the primitive nasal cavity and primary choana

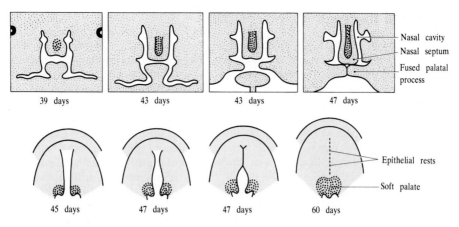

Fig. 1-C Development of the secondary palate
Upper: Frontal sections of the middle part of the lateral palatine processes. **Lower:** Intraoral view of the closure of the posterior palate

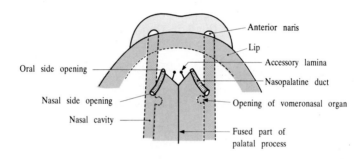

Fig. 1-D Diagram of the transient primordium of the nasopalatine ducts

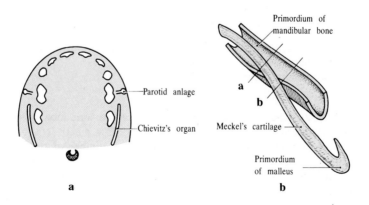

Fig. 1-E
a. Graphic reconstruction of the palate of a newborn infant b. Diagram of the relationship of Meckel's cartilage and the developing mandibular bone.

5

Formation of the Teeth

The development of the teeth requires the presence of three primordial tissues: the enamel organ, the dental papilla and the dental sac or follicle. Together, these three tissues form the tooth germ. The enamel organ, which forms from the oral ectoderm, will give rise to the enamel, the dental papilla will form the dentin and the pulp, and the dental sac will form the cementum, periodontal ligament and the alveolar bone. The dental papilla and the dental follicle arise from ectomesenchyme. During the sixth week, localized histologic changes in the primitive oral ectoderm indicates the beginning of tooth formation. The primitive oral ectoderm proliferates along the crest of the maxillary and mandibular arches to form a horseshoe-shaped band of thickened epithelium. With continued growth, this band of epithelium separates into two parts: the lateral vestibular lamina which forms the labial/buccal vestibule and the lingual dental lamina which will form the teeth (Figs.

functions in the differentiation of odontoblasts for the formation of dentin. In turn, dentin is essential for the continued differentiation of the inner epithelial cells into ameloblasts. The cells of the stratum intermedium are also required for enamel matrix formation since they may form a functional unit with the ameloblasts.

The inner and outer enamel epithelia are continuous with each other at the rim of the enamel organ. This rim is called the cervical loop and represents the presumptive cervix of the future tooth (Fig. 1-19-2). These two epithelia later proliferate to form a bicellular sheath that extends as a skirt around the formative dental pulp. This layer is known as Hertwig's epithelial root sheath (Fig. 1-29-1, Figs. 1-30-1, 2). It is important to note that cells of the stellate reticulum and stratum intermedium are absent from the sheath. The inner layer of the sheath initiates the continued differentiation of odontoblasts for the formation of radicular (root) dentin of the tooth. This sheath may also

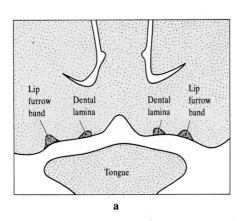
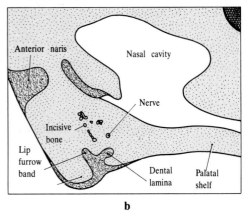

Fig. 1-F Development of the dental lamina and the vestibular lamina
a. 41-day human embryo, frontal section
b. 47-day human embryo, sagittal section

1-6-1, 2; Figs. 1-12-1, 2). The dental lamina continues to enlarge in ten specific locations in each arch for the formation of the primary or deciduous dentition. These epithelial buds proliferate into cap-shaped, then bell-shaped structures referred to as enamel or dental organs (Fig. 1-14-1, 2; Figs. 1-F, G). The enamel organ is separated from the dental papilla by a prominent basement membrane. Histodifferentiation of the enamel organ produces several cellular layers: the outer enamel epithelium, the stellate reticulum, the stratum intermedium and the inner enamel epithelium. The inner enamel epithelium

influence the formation of cementum (Figs. 1-33-1, 2). This sheath is also responsible for the shape and number of roots (Figs. 1-39-1 to 1-42-3). In multirooted teeth, separate partitions extend across the primary apical foramen creating multiple roots (Fig. 1-39-2, Fig. 1-40-1, Fig. 1-41-1, 2; Fig. 1-42-1).

Eruption of the tooth coincides with the appearance of Hertwig's epithelial root sheath. In active eruption, the crown of the tooth moves towards the oral cavity as the root of the tooth lengthens. After the tooth meets its occlusal opponent, crown movement ceases but root

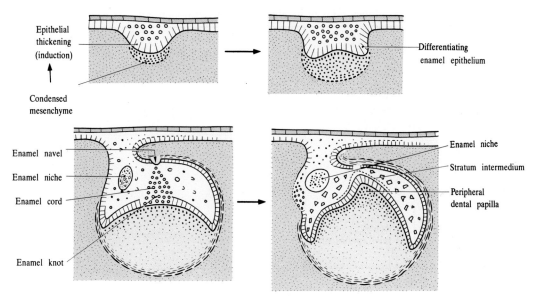

Epithelial
thickening
(induction)

Differentiating
enamel epithelium

Condensed
mesenchyme

Enamel navel

Enamel niche

Enamel cord

Enamel knot

Enamel niche

Stratum intermedium

Peripheral
dental papilla

Fig. 1-G Diagrams of the early development of a tooth

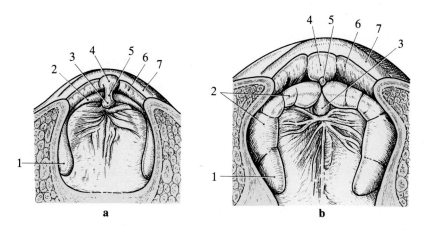

a

b

Fig. 1-H Intraoral view of the lip and palate
a. 3-month fetus **b.** 7-month fetus
1. Developing alveolar ridge **2.** Alveolar ridge **3.** Anterior palatal papilla
4. Superior labial ridge (lip) **5.** Primitive labial frenum (3-month fetus)
Superior labial frenum (7-month fetus) **6.** Oral surface of the lip **7.**
Vermillion border of the lip

formation continues until the anatomic root is completed. The root shape usually tapers from the cementoenamel junction to a blunt point at the root apex where blood vessels and nerves enter through the apical foramen into the root canal (Figs. 1-37-1, 2; Fig. 1-39-1, Fig. 1-40-2, Fig. 1-41-3, Fig. 1-42-2). Multiple accessory canals are also possible.

The eruption of the secondary teeth may be assisted by the presence of a pathway or gubernacular canal through the roof of the bony crypt (Figs. 1-38-1, 2). Epithelial remnants of the dental lamina may be found within the canal. During the process of shedding, the roots of the primary teeth are resorbed as their successor teeth move towards the oral cavity. The roots are resorbed by large multinucleated odontoclasts (Figs. 1-36-1, 2).

The chronology of the development of the primary and secondary dentitions, including eruption and shedding, is given in Tables 1-1, 1-2 and 1-3.

Tabel 1-1 Chronology of Tooth Development

Tooth Number	Dental organ appears	Dentin appears	Primitive alveolus appears
i_1	40 days (in utero)	14 weeks (in utero)	7 weeks (in utero)
i_2	40 days	14 weeks	7 weeks
c	40 days	16 weeks	7 weeks
m_1	43 days	14 weeks	8 weeks
m_2	51 days	18 weeks	10 weeks
I_1	20 weeks (in utero)	3 months (postnatal)	
I_2	20 weeks	10 months	
C	26 weeks	5 months	
P_1	35 weeks	2 years	
P_2	7 months	2 years	
M_1	13 weeks	At birth	
M_2	6 months	2.5 years	
M3	4 years (postnatal)	7 years	

Tabel 1-2 Chronology of Tooth Development

Tooth Number	Completed crown	Emergence into oral cavity	Completed root	
i_1	2 months	6 months (postnatal)	2.5 years	Root formation is completed about 1 to 1.5 years after emergence of the tooth into the oral cavity.
i_2	2 months	7 months	2.5 years	
c	9 months	14 months	3 years	
m_1	6 months	12 months	3 years	
m_2	12 months	20 months	3 years	
I_1	4 years	6 years	9 years	
I_2	5 years	7 years	9 years	
C	6 years	9 years	12 years	Root formation is completed about 2 to 3 years after emergence of the tooth into the oral cavity
P_1	7 years	10 years	13 years	
P_2	7 years	10 years	13 years	
M_1	3 years	6 years	9 years	
M_2	7 years	11 years	14 years	
M3	12 years	19 years	21 years	

Tabel 1-3 Time of Initiation of Root Resorption and Shedding of the Primary Teeth

Tooth Number	Initation of Root Resoption	Shedding of the Primary Teeth
i_1	4 years (postnatal)	6-9 years (postnatal)
i_2	5 years	7-10 years
c	8 years	9-12 years
m_1	6-7 years	10-11 years
m_2	7-8 years	11-12 years

The nasal pit forms from the depression of the nasal placode. The relationship of the maxillary, lateral nasal and medial nasal processes is shown.

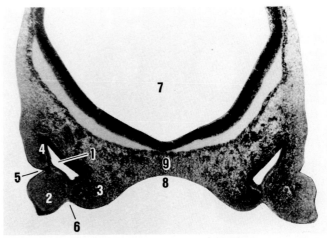

Fig. 1-1-1 Frontal section of the developing face of a 33-day human embryo (10mm CR length). H-E stain X40

The paired swellings of the lower margin of the medial nasal process fuse to form the globular process.

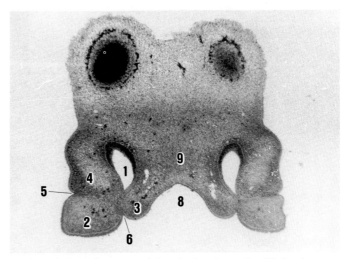

Fig. 1-1-2 Anterior part of developing face of a 35-day human embryo (13mm CR length). X30

1. Nasal pit	**6.** Primitive palatal groove
2. Maxillary process	**7.** Prosencephalon
3. Medial nasal process	**8.** Stomodeum
4. Lateral nasal process	**9.** Roof of oral cavity (frontonasal
5. Nasolacrimal (nasomaxillary groove)	process)

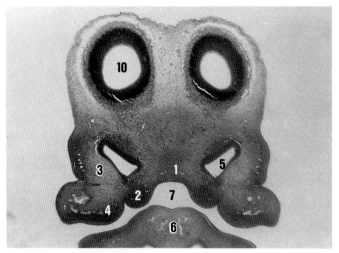

The maxillary process fuses with the medial nasal process. The globular process or intermaxillary segment begins to form with the fusion of the two medial nasal processes.

Fig. 1-2-1 Frontal section of the developing oral cavity of a 35-day human embryo. X30

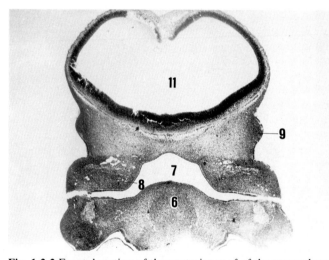

The primordium of the lateral palatine process appears.

Fig. 1-2-2 Frontal section of the posterior roof of the stomodeum in a 35-day human embryo. X30

1. Globular process
2. Medial nasal process
3. Lateral nasal process
4. Maxillary process
5. Anterior nares
6. Mandibular process
7. Stomodeum
8. Region of lateral palatine process
9. Eye
10. Telencephalon
11. Diencephalon

The oronasal membrane ruptures which unites the primary
nasal cavity with the primitive
oral cavity. The stomodeum now
includes the primitive nasal cavity. The nasal septum is beginning
to extend from the frontonasal
process. The tongue is also seen.

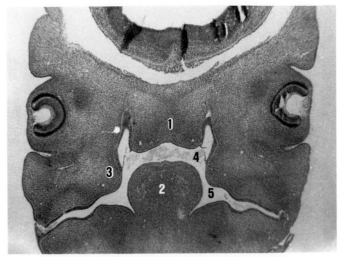

Fig. 1-3-1 Formation of the posterior primary nasal cavity of
a 37-day human embryo. X30

The lateral palatine process
continues to enlarge on either
side of the developing tongue.

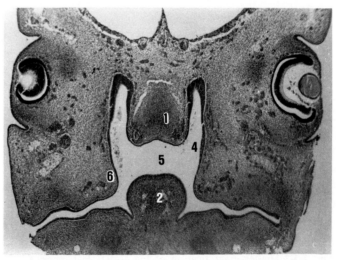

Fig. 1-3-2 Frontal section of the anterior primary nasal cavity
37-day human embryo. X30

1. Nasal septum	**4.**	Posterior nares
2. Tongue	**5.**	Stomodeum
3. Maxillary process	**6.**	Region of the lateral palatine process

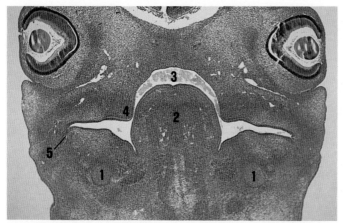

Chievitz's organ, a transient ectodermal outgrowth, appears 4 to 5 days before the primordium of the parotid gland. This organ separates from the surface and usually disappears completely.

Fig. 1-4-1 Frontal section of the middle part of the primitive oral cavity of a 37-day human embryo (16mm CR length). H-E stain X30

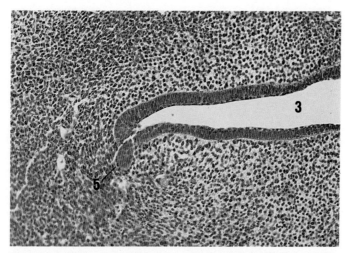

Chievitz's organ appears as an epithelial outgrowth near the corner of the mouth.

Fig. 1-4-2 Higher magnification of Fig. 1-4-1. H-E stain X120

1. Meckel's cartilage
2. Tongue
3. Stomodeum
4. Lateral palatine process
5. Chievitz's organ

Chievitz's organ, before it's dis-
appearance, appears to associate
with the buccal nerve.

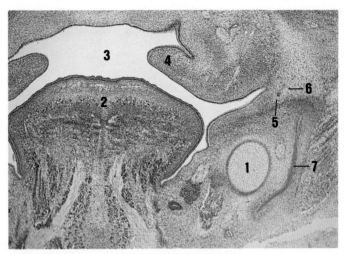

Fig. 1-5-1 Frontal section of the middle part of the primitive
oral cavity of a 45-day human embryo. H-E stain X35

Chievitz's organ is separated
from the oral epithelium and lies
next to the buccal nerve.

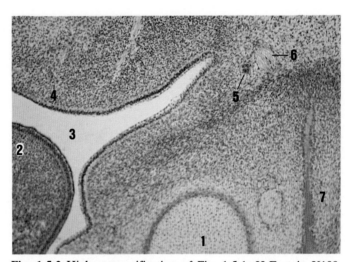

Fig. 1-5-2 Higher magnification of Fig. 1-5-1. H-E stain X100

1. Meckel's cartilage
2. Tongue
3. Stomodeum
4. Lateral palatine process

5. Chievitz's organ
6. Buccal nerve
7. Mandibular bone

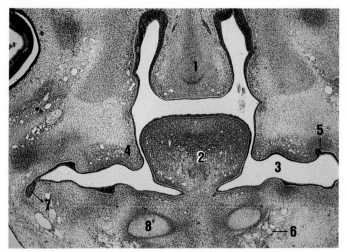

In the 43-day human embryo, the primordium of the parotid gland appears as an epithelial ingrowth from near the corner of the mouth. At this stage of development, the formation of the mandibular bone is just beginning.

Fig. 1-6-1 Frontal section of the middle part of the primitive oral cavity of a 43-day human embryo. H-E stain X30

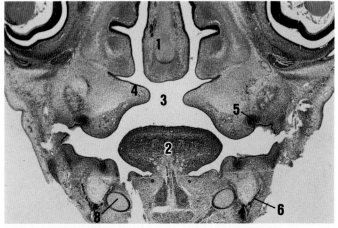

The lateral palatine processes or palatal shelves are in a horizontal orientation. The developing mandibular bone can be seen.

Fig. 1-6-2 Frontal section of the middle part of primitive oral cavity of a 43-day human embryo. H-E stain X14

1. Nasal septum	5. Tooth germ (m1)
2. Tongue	6. Mandibular bone
3. Stomodeum	7. Primordium of parotid gland
4. Lateral palatine process	8. Meckel's cartilage

The anterior portion of the lateral palatine processes grow towards the midline to contact each other and the primary palate.

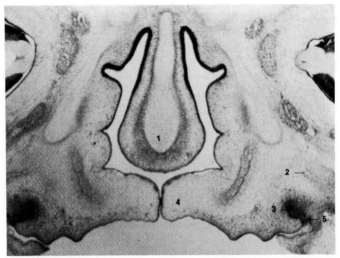

Fig. 1-7-1 Frontal section of the middle part of a forming secondary palate of a 47-day human embryo. X27

The anterior parts of the secondary palate are fused. See Fig. 13-A for the development of incisive and maxillary bones.

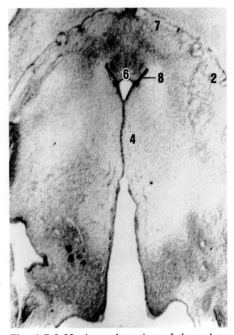

Fig. 1-7-2 Horizontal section of the palate of a 47-day human embryo. X36

1.	Nasal septum	5.	Vestibular lamina
2.	Maxillary bone	6.	Primary palate
3.	Dental lamina	7.	Incisive bone
4.	Lateral palatine process	8.	Primordium of nasopalatine duct

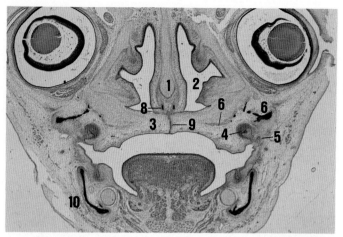

The lateral palatine processes and the nasal septum fuse with each other. The intervening epithelium within the processes disintegrates into epithelial rests.

Fig. 1-8-1 Frontal section of the middle part of secondary palate of a 47-day human embryo (32mm CR length). H-E stain X10

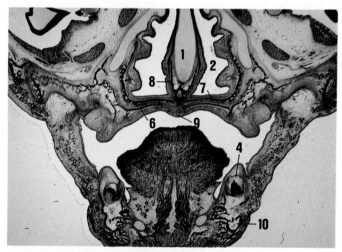

Epithelial rests that persist within the fused palatine processes may form epithelial pearls.

Fig. 1-8-2 Frontal section of the middle part of secondary palate of an 11-week human fetus (71mm CR length). Azan stain X6.5

1.	Nasal septum	**6.**	Maxillary bone
2.	Nasal cavity	**7.**	Palatine bone
3.	Lateral palatine process	**8.**	Vomer bone
4.	Tooth germ (m1)	**9.**	Epithelial rest
5.	Vestibular lamina	**10.**	Mandibular bone

Primitive nasopalatine ducts undergo canalization in the 13-week human fetus.

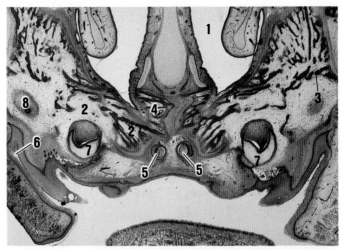

Fig. 1-9-1 Frontal section of the palate of a 13-week human fetus. H-E stain X10

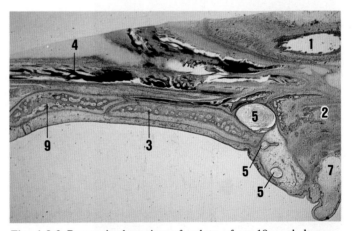

Fig. 1-9-2 Parasagittal section of palate of an 18-week human fetus. Masson stain X10

1. Nasal cavity
2. Incisive bone
3. Maxillary bone
4. Vomer bone
5. Nasopalatine duct
6. Lip furrow
7. Tooth germ of primary lateral incisor
8. Tooth germ of primary canine
9. Palatine bone

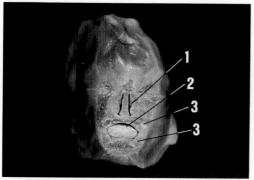
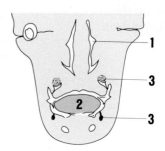

Fig. 1-10-1 Frontal section of the head of a 3-month human fetus.

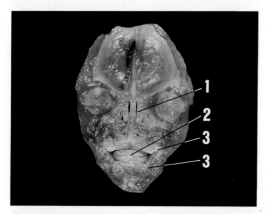
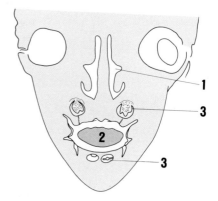

Fig. 1-10-2 Frontal section of the head of a 6-month human fetus.

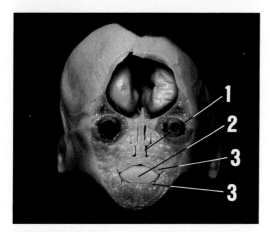
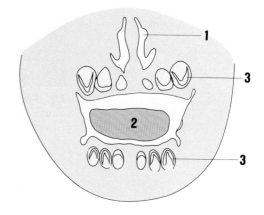

Fig. 1-10-3 Frontal section of the head of a 10-month human fetus.

1. Nasal cavity   **2.** Tongue   **3.** Tooth germ

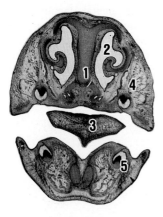

Fig. 1-11-1 Frontal section through the head of an ape fetus.

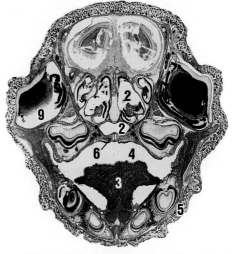

Fig. 1-11-2 Frontal section through the head of an ape fetus.

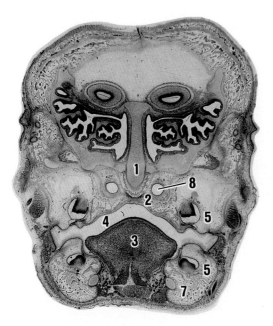

Fig. 1-11-3 Frontal section through the head of an ape fetus.

1.	Nasal septum	**6.**	Palate
2.	Nasal cavity	**7.**	Meckel's cartilage
3.	Tongue	**8.**	Sphenoid sinus
4.	Oral cavity	**9.**	Eye
5.	Tooth germ		

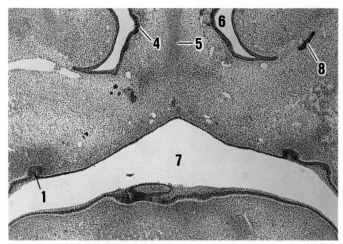

Fig. 1-12-1 Frontal section of the development of the tooth germ of a 41-day human embryo (20mm CR length). H-E stain X20

The dental lamina for the deciduous or primary teeth develop as bud-shaped epithelial extensions from the dental band. These buds enlarge to form the enamel organ.

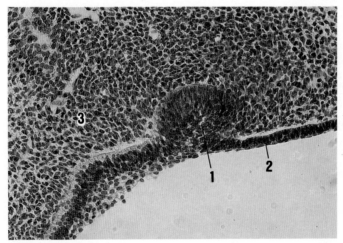

Fig. 1-12-2 Higher magnification of part of Fig. 1-12-1 showing developing tooth in the bud stage. H-E stain X600

1. Tooth bud of primary lateral incisor
2. Oral epithelium
3. Mesenchymal connective tissue (lamina propria)
4. Primordium of vomeronasal organ (Jacobson's organ)
5. Primitive septal cartilage
6. Nasal cavity
7. Oral cavity
8. Primordium of nasolacrimal duct

The dental lamina for the deciduous or primary teeth develop as bud-shaped epithelial extensions from the dental band. These buds enlarge to form the enamel organ.

Development of a provisional alveolar ridge which disappears as the maxilla grows. Also refer to Fig. 1-H.

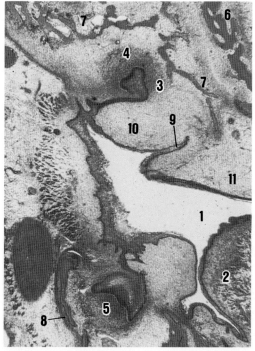

Fig. 1-13-1 Frontal section of an 11-week human fetus (70mm CR length). H-E stain X80

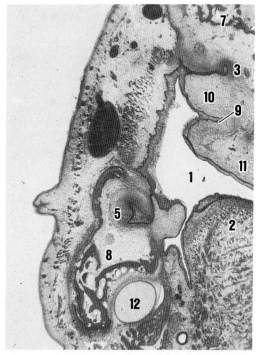

Fig. 1-13-2 Frontal section of an 11-week human fetus. H-E stain X80

1. Oral cavity
2. Tongue
3. Tooth germ of primary second molar
4. Dental sac or dental follicle
5. Tooth germ of primary first molar
6. Palatine bone
7. Maxillary bone
8. Mandibular bone
9. Temporary epithelial groove
10. Provisional alveolar ridge
11. Palate
12. Meckel's cartilage

The cells of the stellate reticulum near the inner enamel epithelium proliferate to form a transient structure called the enamel knot.

The cells of the enamel knot continue to proliferate to form the transient enamel cord which extends to the enamel navel. They form at the site of the future cusp tip or incisal edge.

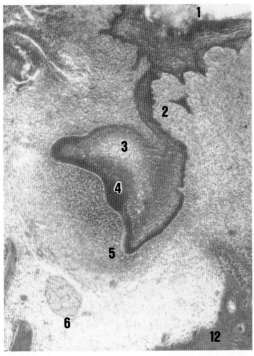

Fig. 1-14-1 Higher magnification of section similar to Fig. 1-13-1. H-E stain X200

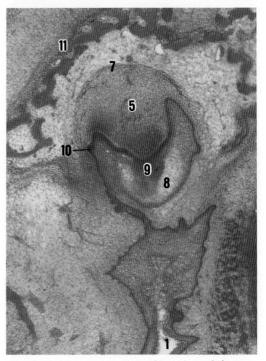

Fig. 1-14-2 Frontal section of an 11-week human fetus (70mm CR length). H-E stain X200

1. Oral cavity
2. Dental lamina
3. Enamel organ of primary second molar
4. Enamel knot
5. Dental papilla
6. Inferior alveolar nerve
7. Dental sac or dental follicle
8. Enamel organ of primary first molar
9. Enamel cord
10. Successional dental lamina
11. Maxillary bone
12. Mandibular bone

Infolding of the outer enamel epithelium at the enamel navel brings blood vessels in the mesenchyme closer to the cells of the enamel cord.

The cells in the center of the enamel organ produce hydrophilic proteoglycans which, with the influx of water, separates them from each other. The cells become stellate-shaped. This region is called the stellate reticulum.

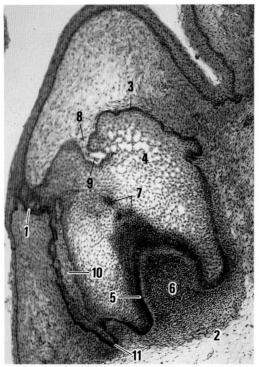

Fig. 1-15-1 Frontal section of primary canine tooth germ of a 13-week human fetus. H-E stain X180

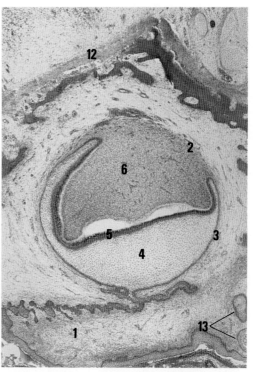

Fig. 1-15-2 Frontal section of a primary lateral incisor tooth germ. H-E stain X190

1.	Dental lamina	**8.**	Enamel navel
2.	Dental sac or follicle	**9.**	Blood vessel
3.	Outer enamel epithelium	**10.**	Enamel niche
4.	Stellate reticulum	**11.**	Successional dental lamina
5.	Inner enamel epithelium	**12.**	Incisive bone
6.	Dental papilla	**13.**	Nasopalatine duct
7.	Enamel cord		

A fibrovascular membranous structure, the dental follicle, surrounds the enamel organ and the dental papilla. Cells of the follicle will produce cementum and the periodontal ligament. Mesenchymal proliferation produces depressions on the mesial and distal sides of the dental lamina known as the enamel niche. The successional dental lamina also appears at this time.

The continued expansion of the enamel niche divides the dental lamina into a medial and lateral lamina. The latter is the first to disappear.

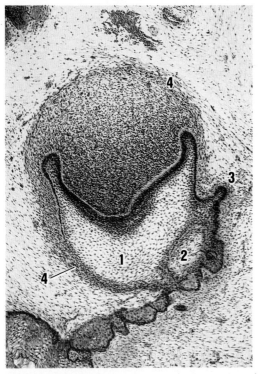

Fig. 1-16-1 Frontal section of the tooth germ of a primary lateral incisor of an 11-week human fetus. H-E stain X200

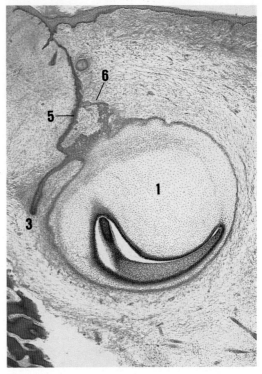

Fig. 1-16-2 Frontal section of the tooth germ of a primary first molar of an 18-week human fetus. H-E stain X140

1. Stellate reticulum (enamel pulp)
2. Enamel niche
3. Successional dental lamina
4. Dental sac or dental follicle
5. Medial dental lamina
6. Lateral dental lamina

Frontal sections near the primary central incisor tooth buds often sections the incisive or palatine papilla. However, in this section the labial frenum is seen.

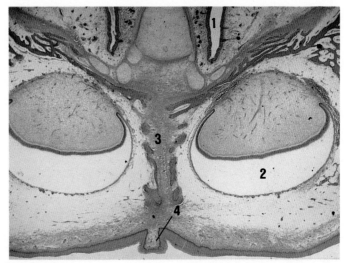

Fig. 1-17-1 Frontal section of a 14-week human fetus. H-E stain X76

Epithelial rests derived from the disintegration of the dental lamina may form epithelial pearls.

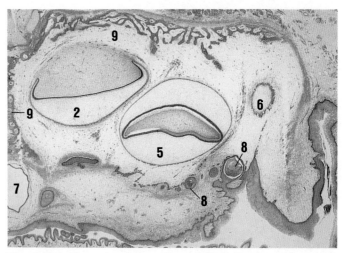

Fig. 1-17-2 Frontal section of a 14-week human fetus. H-E stain X57

1. Nasal cavity
2. Enamel organ of primary central incisor
3. Incisive canal
4. Labial frenum
5. Enamel organ of primary lateral incisor
6. Enamel organ of primary canine or cuspid
7. Nasopalatine duct
8. Epithelial pearl
9. Incisive bone

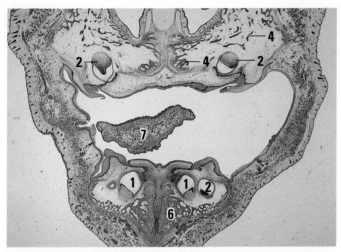

Fig. 1-18-1 15-week human fetus. Frontal section of head. H-E stain X11

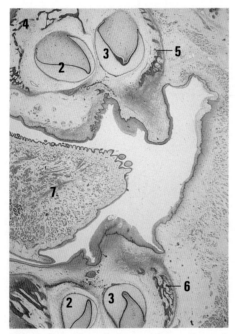

Fig. 1-18-2 17-week human fetus. Frontal section of head. H-E stain X13

1. Enamel organ of primary central incisor
2. Enamel organ of primary lateral incisor
3. Enamel organ of primary canine
4. Incisive bone
5. Maxillary bone
6. Mandibular bone
7. Tongue

The initial site of hard tissue matrix formation and mineralization is in the center of the incisal edge. Mineralization then extends to the mesial and distal ridges. Enamel formation begins after dentin has been deposited.

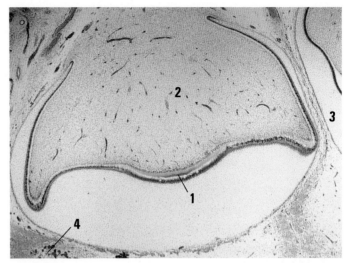

Fig. 1-19-1 Frontal section of maxilla showing the initial calcification of a tooth germ. H-E stain X200

The rim of the enamel organ, where the inner enamel epithelium loops around to join the outer enamel epithelium, is called the cervical loop.

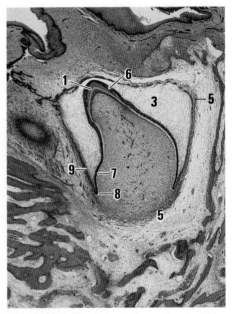

Fig. 1-19-2 Frontal section of mandible. H-E stain X53

1. Dentin
2. Immature pulp of primary lateral incisor
3. Enamel organ of primary canine
4. Epithelial rests of dental lamina
5. Dental sac or dental follicle
6. Enamel
7. Inner enamel epithelium
8. Cervical loop
9. Outer enamel epithelium

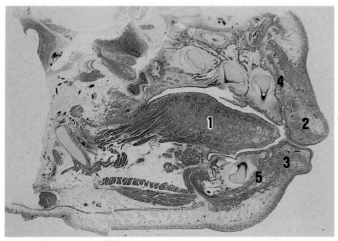

Fig. 1-20-1 Sagittal section through the head of a human fetus. H-E stain X11

1. Tongue, 2. Upper lip, 3. Lower lip, 4.Maxillary tooth germ, 5. Mandibular tooth germ

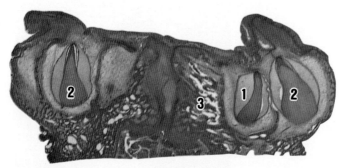

Fig. 1-20-2 Frontal section through mandible of a human fetus. H-E stain X18

1. Tooth germ of primary lateral incisor, 2. Tooth germ of primary canine, 3. Mandibular bone

Initiation of enamel and dentin
formation during the morphologic
bell stage.

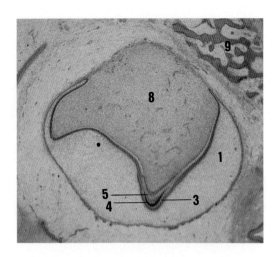

Fig. 1-21-1 Frontal section of the maxilla
showing the initial calcification of enamel
and dentin in the primary first molar
tooth. H-E stain X60

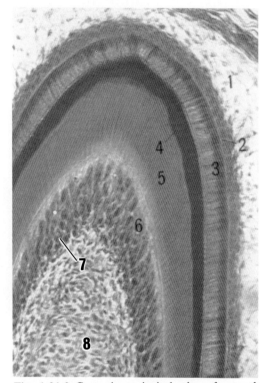

Fig. 1-21-2 Cusp tip or incisal edge of a tooth
showing the early formation of enamel. H-E
stain X600

1. Stellate reticulum
2. Stratum intermedium
3. Ameloblast
4. Enamel
5. Dentin

6. Odontoblast
7. Cell-rich zone of immature pulp
8. Cells of the immature pulp
9. Maxilla

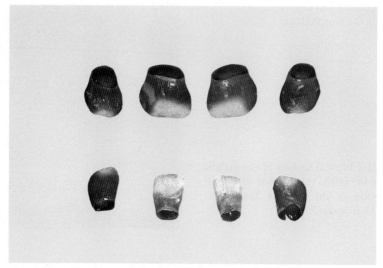

Fig. 1-22-1 Crowns of incompletely-formed incisor teeth

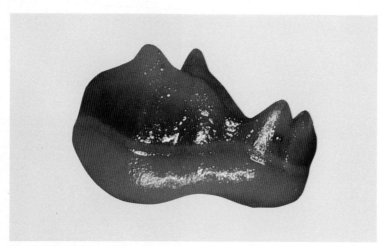

Fig. 1-22-2 Crown of an immature molar tooth.

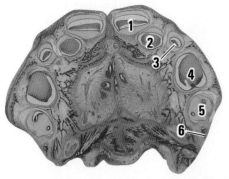

Fig. 1-23-1 Horizontal section of maxilla of a 5-month human fetus. H-E stain

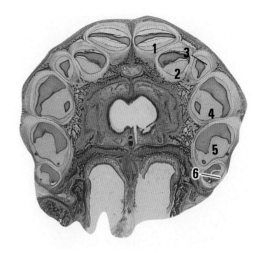

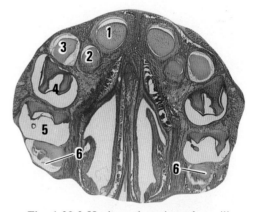

Fig. 1-23-2 Horizontal section of maxilla of a 6-month human fetus. H-E stain

1. Primary central incisor tooth germ
2. Primary lateral incisor tooth germ
3. Primary canine tooth germ
4. Primary first molar tooth germ
5. Primary second molar tooth germ
6. Secondary first molar tooth germ

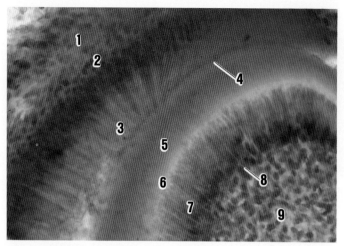

A cell-rich zone of immature, spindle-shaped cells lies between the odontoblasts and the cells of the immature pulp.

Fig. 1-24-1 Developing crown of a tooth germ. H-E stain X800

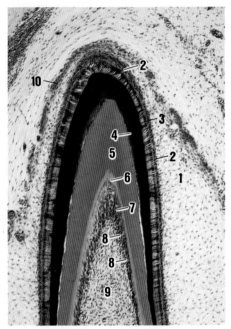

The cells of the stratum intermedium form a 2-to-3 cell thick layer between the stellate reticulum and the ameloblasts.

Fig. 1-24-2 Crown of an incisor tooth germ. H-E stain X360

1. Stellate reticulum	6. Predentin
2. Stratum intermedium	7. Odontoblast
3. Ameloblast	8. Cell-rich zone
4. Enamel	9. Pulp cells
5. Dentin	10. Outer enamel epithelium

With the initiation of hard tissue formation, the distance between the outer enamel epithelium and the ameloblasts is reduced. The outer enamel epithelium also becomes highly infolded with capillaries. This facilitates the exchange of materials between the blood and the cells of stratum intermedium and the ameloblast.

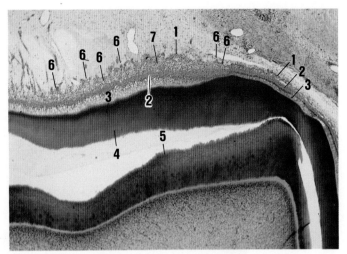

Fig. 1-25-1 Crown of primary lateral incisor tooth germ. H-E stain X360

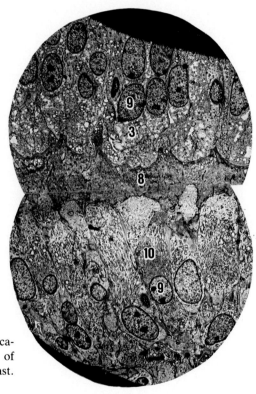

Fig. 1-25-2 Higher magnification electron micrograph of ameloblast and odontoblast. X2,000

1.	Outer enamel epithelium	**6.**	Blood vessel
2.	Stratum intermedium	**7.**	Stellate reticulum
3.	Ameloblast	**8.**	Predentin
4.	Enamel	**9.**	Cell nucleus
5.	Dentin	**10.**	Odontoblast

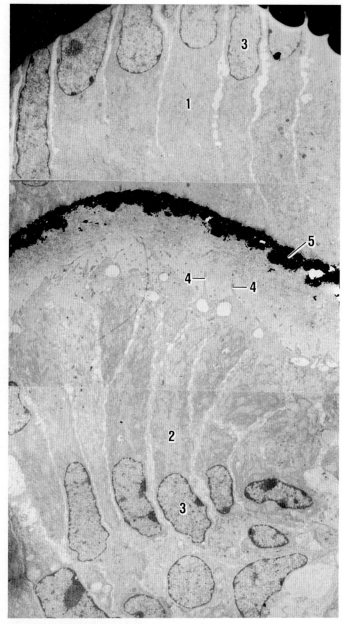

Fig. 1-26 Composite electron micrograph of odontogenic cells in the rat tooth during initial dentin formation. X2,600

1. Ameloblast
2. Odontoblast
3. Cell nucleus
4. Odontoblast process (Tomes' dentinal fiber)
5. Dentin

Odontoblast processes extend into the predentin from the main cell body of the odontoblast. Evidence of branching of the processes can be seen.

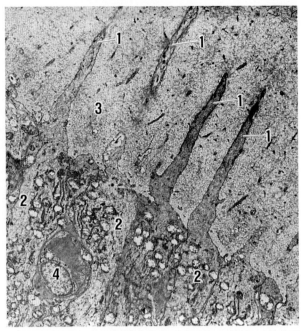

Fig. 1-27-1 Electron micrograph of an odontoblast. X4,000

Odontoblasts are tall columnar cells that line the surface of the predentin. The odontoblast processes are not evident in this section.

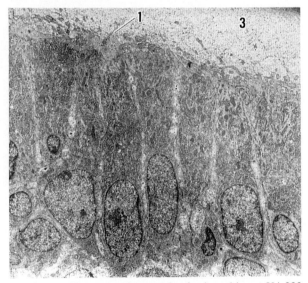

Fig. 1-27-2 Electron micrograph of odontoblasts. X4,000

1. Odontoblast process (Tomes')
2. Odontoblast
3. Predentin
4. Nucleus of endothelial cell

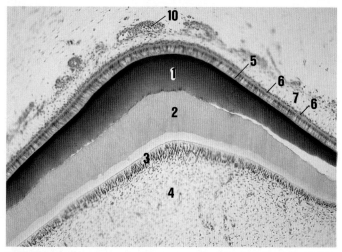

Fig. 1-28-1 Cusp tip of a molar tooth germ. H-E stain X400

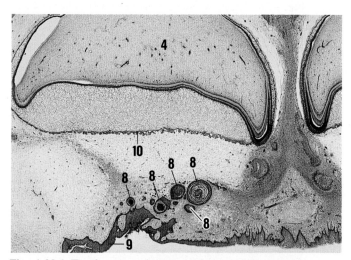

Fig. 1-28-2 Tooth germ of central incisor. H-E stain X144

Remnants of the dental lamina have become epithelial pearls which are characterized by their onion-like structure. The central region of the pearl is keratinized.

1. Enamel	**6.** Stratum intermedium
2. Dentin	**7.** Stellate reticulum
3. Odontoblast	**8.** Remnants of dental lamina
4. Dental pulp	**9.** Oral epithelium
5. Ameloblast	**10.** Outer enamel epithelium

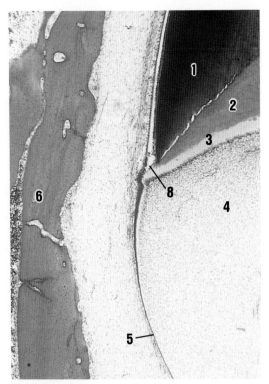

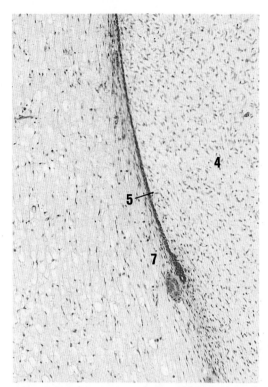

Fig. 1-29-1 Region near the cervix of the tooth of a molar tooth germ. H-E stain X132

Fig. 1-29-2 Cervical extension of the enamel organ for root formation is called Hertwig's epithelial root sheath. van Gieson X264

1.	Enamel	**5.**	Epithelial root sheath
2.	Dentin	**6.**	Alveolar bone
3.	Predentin	**7.**	Dental follicle
4.	Dental pulp	**8.**	Cervical margin

The region near the cervical margin of the tooth still may retain some cells of the stellate reticulum.

The perifollicular region beneath developing root shows vacuolar degeneration and pyknotic cells (arrows).

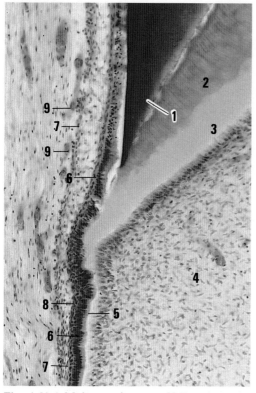

Fig. 1-30-1 Molar tooth germ. H-E stain X132

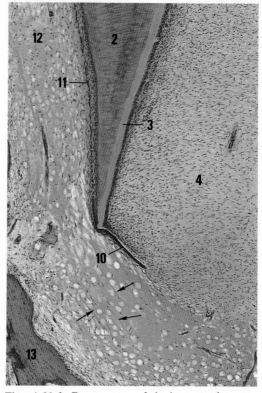

Fig. 1-30-2 Root area of incisor tooth. van Gieson stain X132

1. Enamel
2. Dentin
3. Predentin
4. Immature pulp
5. Ameloblast
6. Stratum intermedium
7. Outer enamel epithelium
8. Stellate reticulum
9. Blood vessel
10. Epithelial root diaphragm
11. Epithelial rest of Malassez
12. Periodontal ligament
13. Alveolar bone

The terminal portion of Hertwig's epithelial root sheath will form a tapering tooth root. The terminal portion has been called the apical loop.

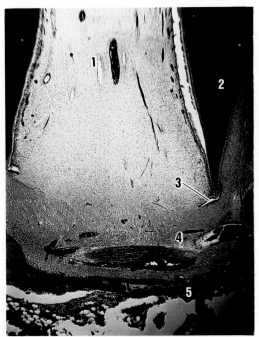

Fig. 1-31-1 Primary apical foramen (radicular area) of incisor tooth germ.

1. Dental pulp 2. Dentin 3. Epithelial diaphragm 4. Dental follicle 5. Alveolar bone

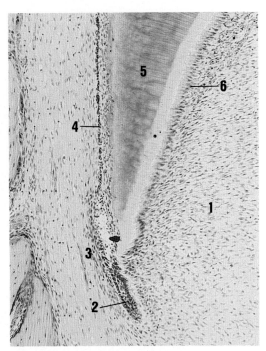

Fig. 1-31-2 Hertwig's epithelial root sheath composed of a bicellular layer of cells.

1. Dental pulp 2. Epithelial root sheath
3. Dental follicle 4. Epithelial rest of Malassez
5. Dentin 6. Odontoblast

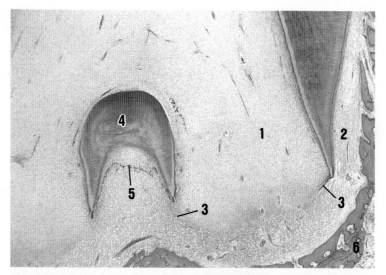

Fig. 1-32-1 Root formation of a multirooted tooth showing Hertwig's epithelial root sheath. H-E stain X200

1. Dental pulp 2. Periodontal ligament 3. Epithelial diaphragm 4. Dentin of root furcation 5. Epithelial rest of Malassez 6. Alveolar bone

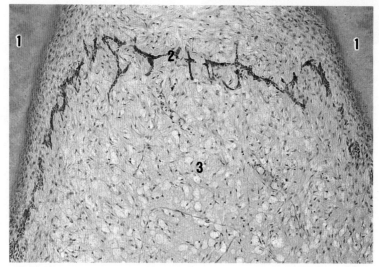

Fig. 1-32-2 Tangential section of the furcation between the roots of a multirooted tooth. H-E stain X400

1. Dentin 2. Epithelial rest of Malassez 3. Periodontal ligament

Cementogenesis begins shortly after the formation of Hertwig's epithelial root sheath. Cementum is deposited on the newly-formed layer of root dentin by cementoblasts. Cementoblasts differentiate from the inner region of the dental follicle.

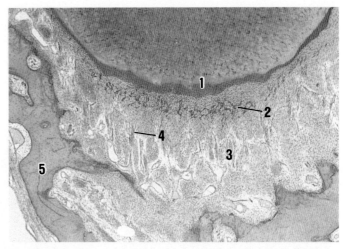

Fig. 1-33-1 Tangential section of apical periodontal ligament space. H-E stain X290

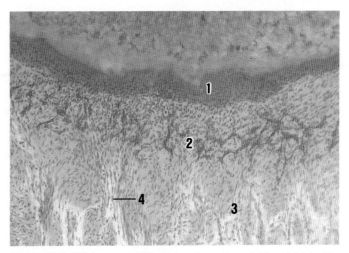

Fig. 1-33-2 Higher magnification of a part of Fig. 1-31-1. H-E stain X390

1. Cementum
2. Epithelial rest of Malassez
3. Periodontal ligament
4. Periodontal ligament principal fiber bundle
5. Alveolar bone

The relationship of the primary tooth and the secondary successor tooth is seen. Each successor tooth is located apical and lingual to the primary tooth it will replace. This position is especially true for the incisor teeth.

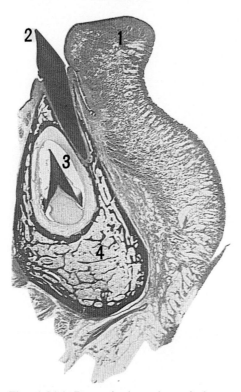

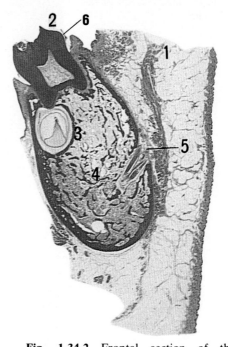

Fig. 1-34-1 Parasagittal section of the mandible. H-E stain
1. Lower lip 2. Primary incisor 3. Secondary or permanent tooth germ 4. Mandible

Fig. 1-34-2 Frontal section of the mandible. H-E stain
1. Cheek 2. Primary or deciduous molar tooth 3. Secondary or permanent tooth germ 4. Mandible 5. Mental foramen with mental nerve 6. Oral debris

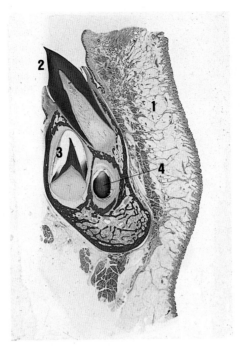

Fig. 1-35-1 Frontal section of anterior mandible showing primary teeth and the successor teeth. H-E stain

1. Cheek 2. Primary canine 3. Secondary successor 4. Secondary first premolar

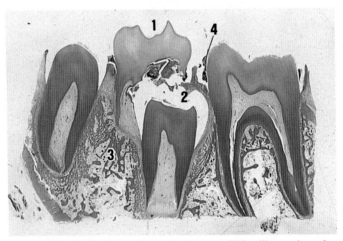

Fig. 1-35-2 Sagittal section of the mandible illustrating the eruption of the secondary premolar. H-E stain

1. Primary second molar 2. Secondary second premolar 3. Alveolar bone 4. Interproximal debris

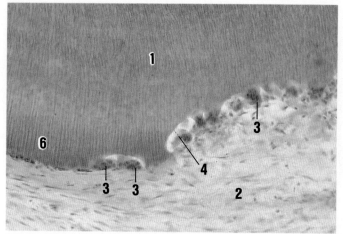

During the resorption of a primary tooth, the nerves and blood vessels of the pulp degenerate along with the odontoblasts and the connective tissue cells and fibers.

Fig. 1-36-1 Resorption of the dentin of a primary tooth. H-E stain X112

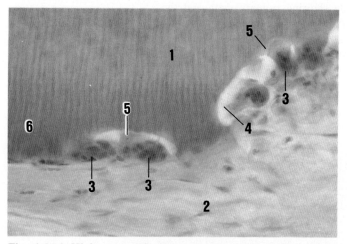

During periods of active root resorption, odontoclasts resorb the dentin. These active cells reside within depressions of the root surface or Howship's lacunae. During quiescent periods, odontoclasts are not seen within the lacunae.

Fig. 1-36-2 Higher magnification of part of Fig. 1-36-1. H-E stain X448

1. Dentin	**4.** Howship's lacuna
2. Dental pulp	**5.** Ruffled border
3. Odontoclast	**6.** Secondary dentin

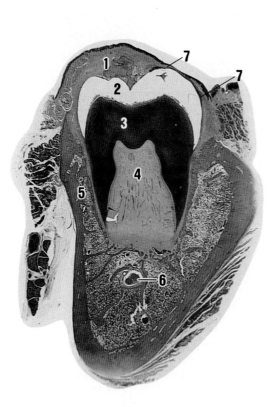

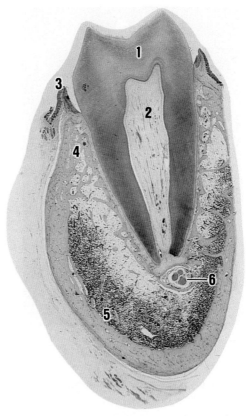

Fig. 1-37-1 Secondary molar during active eruption showing a wide open apical foramen. The relationship with the mandibular canal should be noted. H-E stain

1. Oral mucosa 2. Decalcified enamel (space) 3. Predentin 4. Dental pulp 5. Alveolar bone 6. Mandibular canal with inferior alveolar neurovascular bundle 7. Reduced enamel epithelium

Fig. 1-37-2 Newly erupted secondary molar tooth. H-E stain

1. Dentin 2. Dental pulp 3. Gingiva 4. Alveolar bone 5. Mandibular bone 6. Mandibular canal with inferior alveolar neurovascular bundle

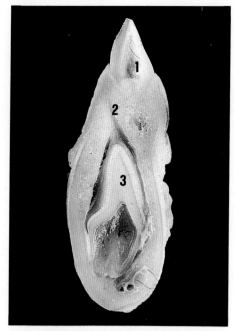

Fig. 1-38-1 Longitudinal section of the mandible showing the eruption of a successional tooth.

1. Primary canine 2. Gubernacular canal 3. Secondary canine

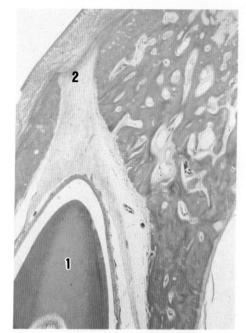

Fig. 1-38-2 Detail of the gubernacular canal during eruption of a secondary tooth. Azan stain

1. Secondary canine crown 2. Gubernacular canal

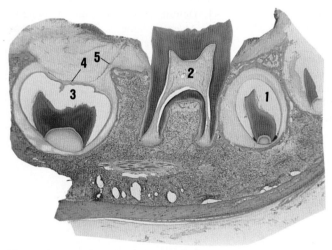

The accessional dental lamina for the secondary molar tooth buds is a distal extension of the dental lamina of the primary second molar.

Fig. 1-38-3 Mandible in a stage of tooth replacement (Sagittal section). H-E stain

1. Tooth germ of the secondary second premolar 2. Secondary first molar 3. Tooth germ of the secondary second molar 4. Reduced enamel epithelium 5. Epithelial rest of accessional dental lamina

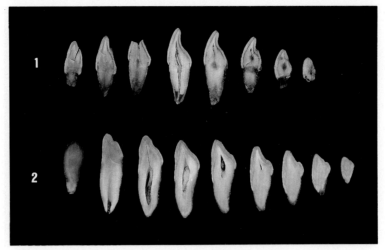

Fig. 1-39-1 Longitudinal 1mm thick serial mesial-distal ground sections.
1. Maxillary central incisor 2. Maxillary canine

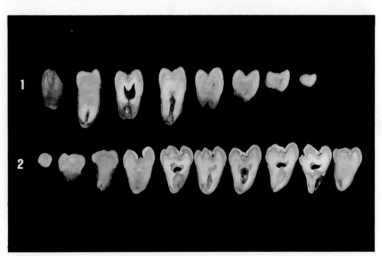

Fig. 1-39-2 1mm Serial mesial-distal ground sections.
1. Maxillary premolar 2. Maxillary third molar

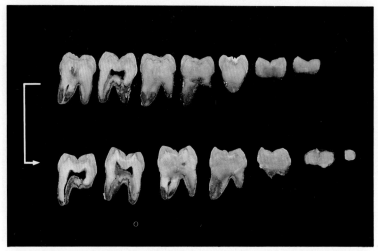

Fig. 1-40-1 Longitudinal 1mm thick serial mesial-distal ground sections. Maxillary first molar

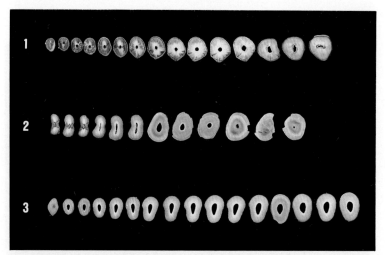

Fig. 1-40-2 Transverse 1mm thick serial ground sections.
1. Maxillary canine 2. Mandibular premolar 3. Maxillary premolar

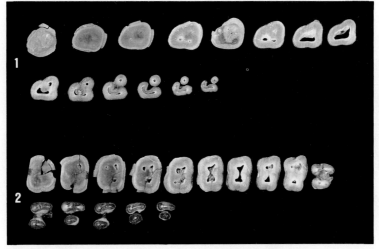

Fig. 1-41-1 Transverse 1mm thick serial ground sections.
1. Maxillary second molar 2. Maxillary first molar

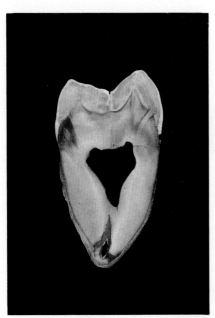

Fig. 1-41-2 Frontal ground section of the maxillary third molar.

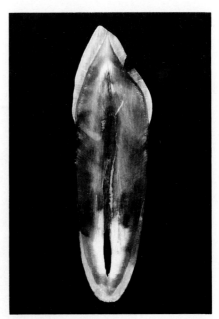

Fig. 1-41-3 Sagittal ground section of the maxillary canine.

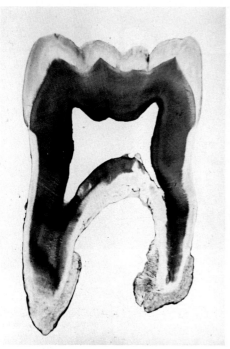

Fig. 1-42-1 Mesial-distal ground section of the mandibular first molar. Carbol-fuchsin stain

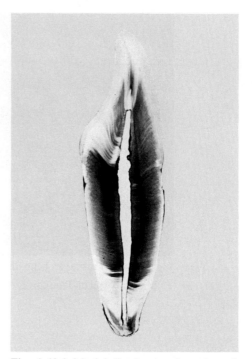

Fig. 1-42-2 Mesial-distal ground section of the maxillary central incisor. Carbol-fuchsin stain

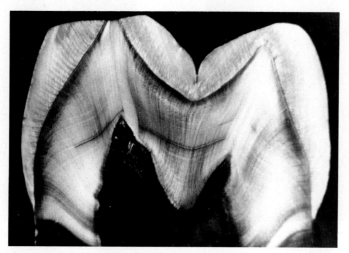

Fig. 1-42-3 Buccal-lingual ground section of the maxillary molar crown.

2
Tooth Structure: Enamel

Tooth Structure: Enamel

Human enamel is the hardest substance in the body and a poor conductor of both heat and electricity. It is composed of inorganic materials (96-98%) and organic substances including water (2-4%). These percentages will vary with location in the crown and the age of the tooth. The inorganic content consists of a crystalline calcium phosphate known as hydroxyapatite. Hydroxyapatite is also found in dentin, cementum, bone and calcified cartilage. The organic material consists of the proteins enamelin and amelogenin. The enamel is thickest at the crest of cusps or incisal edges (up to 2.5mm). It becomes thinner within the fissures and pits of multicuspid teeth and over the facial, lingual and interproximal surfaces, where it tapers to a minimal thickness (less than 100 μm) at the cervical margin (Figs. 2-A, B; Figs. 1-41-2, 3; Figs. 1-42-1, 3; Fig. 2-1-1). The enamel is harder, or more mineralized, at the surface than it is closer to the dentin. Mature enamel cannot be regenerated nor repaired due to the lack of formative cells, the ameloblasts. The histological examination of enamel requires the use of ground sections of the tooth. Since enamel is about 96% mineral, it is lost during normal decalcification procedures.

The basic structural component of enamel is called an enamel rod. The rods originate at the dentinoenamel junction and extend through the thickness of the enamel to the surface. In the inner one-third to one-half of the enamel, the rods are in groups with a wavy arrangement, but in the outer layers they are straighter and reach the surface where the enamel rods are generally oriented perpendicular to a tangent at the surface of the crown (Fig. 2-C: a). Overall, the enamel rods follow a complicated, undulating S-shaped course from the dentinoenamel junction toward the surface. This pattern is best illustrated by examining thin, mid-coronal, transverse discs cut parallel to the general direction of the rods. Within each disc, the enamel rods generally lie perpendicular to the dentinoenamel junction as

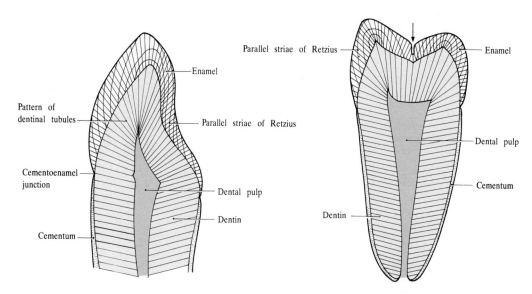

Fig. 2-A Diagram of a longitudinal labial-lingual section of an incisor. The enamel is thicker on labial side of the crown. The thickness is reduced towards the cervical margin.

Fig. 2-B Diagram of a longitudinal mesial-distal section of a maxillary premolar. The deep central fissure (arrow) is prone to caries formation.

they begin their path towards the surface. After a short distance, they turn in a plane horizontal to their long axis, first in one direction then in the other. This occurs several times before they assume a straight alignment towards the surface. The rods in those discs just above or below course in just the opposite fashion (Fig. 2-8-2). In the cervical region of the crown, the enamel rods may be directed apically or appear to have a different arrangement (Fig. 2-C: b).

A ground section cut obliquely across the cusp or incisal edge near the dentin will demonstrate the tortuous pathways of the rods sometimes referred to "gnarled" enamel (Fig. 2-2-1).

The Enamel Rod

The enamel rod is formed by four ameloblasts. The diameter of the single rod is smallest at the dentinoenamel junction and increases towards the surface. The average diameter of the rod is about 4 μm. The number of enamel rods is estimated at 40,000/mm^2 at the surface, while there are about 44,000/mm^2 near the dentinoenamel junction. If the rod is cut perpendicular to its long axis, the most common shape seems to be that of an arcade or a key-hole (Fig. 2D: b). However, the shape of the rod will vary with the plane of section and the location of the rod within the enamel (Fig. 2-D).

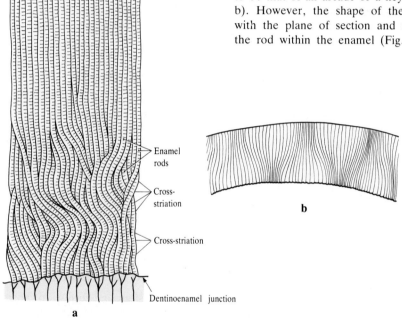

a

b

Enamel rods

Cross-striation

Cross-striation

Dentinoenamel junction

Fig. 2-C Diagram of the arrangement of the enamel rods.
a. Diagram of a ground section of the mid-coronal region in a molar crown aligned with the enamel rods. **b.** Diagram of a ground section of the cervical region in a canine crown aligned with the enamel rods illustrating the variation in rod arrangement.

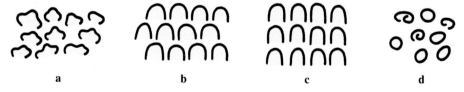

a b c d

Fig. 2-D Diagram of the various shapes of the enamel rods in different regions of the crown.
a. Near the outer surface **b.** About 100 μm from the dentinoenamel junction **c.** About 50 μm from the dentinoenamel junction **d.** Near the dentinoenamel junction

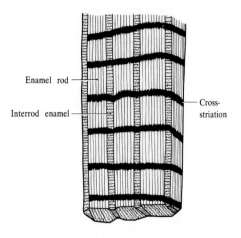

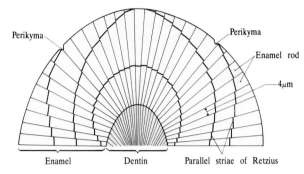

Fig. 2-E Diagram of enamel rods

Fig. 2-F Diagram of the relation between the enamel rods and the lines or striae of Retzius.

Cross-Striations of Enamel Rods

Enamel is formed in a rhythmic manner. The amount of enamel matrix produced in a 24-hour period is marked by a dark line or cross-striation of the rod. In longitudinal sections of enamel rods, these cross-striations appear at intervals of about 4 μm (Fig. 2-3-1, Figs. 2-5-1, 2, 3). In scanning electron micrographs, these cross-striations are represented by variations in the thickness or width of the rods, appearing as dilations or varicosities (Figs. 2-5-1, 2, 3). These lines correspond to the daily pattern of enamel rod formation (Fig. 2-E).

Interrod Enamel

As mentioned, the most common appearance of the enamel rods cut perpendicular to their long axis in the mid-coronal region of the crown is a key-hole shape (Fig. 2-6-1). The enamel rod, in this view, can be divided into two parts: the rod head and rod tail (Fig. 2-D: b; Fig. 2-6-2). The heads are usually towards the occlusal surface and are separated by about 1 μm of interrod enamel or the tails. The nature of the inorganic material within the rod head and rod tail is the same. There is, however, a difference in the orientation of the hydroxyapatite crystals. The crystals within the head are aligned parallel to the long axis of the rod and those within the tail deviate from parallel (Fig. 2-6-2, Figs. 2-7-1, 2, 3). In a different plane of section, the interrod enamel and the enamel rod heads flow together making the transition more difficult to visualize (Fig. 2-D: a, c, d; Fig. 2-9-3, Fig. 2-12-2).

Enamel Rod Sheath

Within enamel, the junction of an enamel head and an adjacent tail represents an interrod space lined by hydroxyapatite crystals with greatly different patterns of orientation (Figs. 2-7-2, 3). This space contains considerable organic matrix and water. There is a slightly greater amount of organic matrix at the convex border around the top of the enamel rod between the rod and interrod enamel. This region or interface is called the enamel rod sheath (Fig. 2-D, Fig. 2-4-2, Fig. 2-6-2).

Lines or Striae of Retzius

Longitudinal ground sections of enamel have brown parallel lines of different widths and are termed lines or striae of Retzius. When viewed in a transverse section of the crown, the lines are seen as parallel concentric circles similar to growth rings on a tree (Fig. 2-F). The brown striae contain more organic matrix than the adjacent lighter areas. The appositional pattern of enamel growth is illustrated by a series of these brown lines. During tooth formation, the first layer of enamel is deposited as the dentinoenamel junction under what will become the cusp tip or incisal edge. The process of deposition of enamel matrix continues in a wave-like manner towards the cervical loop until the last enamel is deposited as the cervical margin. In a longitudinal ground section, these light to dark brown lines begin at the dentinoenamel junction and arch obliquely upward and outward to the surface of the enamel (Fig. 2-F, Fig. 2-3-1, Figs. 2-9-1, 2, 3). The enamel rods within

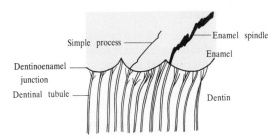

Fig. 2-G Diagram of the relation between the dentinal tubules and the simple and bulbous forms of enamel spindles.

a line are hypomineralized with an increase in organic material and may show an irregular arrangement (Fig. 2-9-3). The cross-striations of these enamel rods are also accentuated (Fig. 2-3-1). The lines of Retzius are normally present in teeth, however, disease and nutritional changes will increase the number and width of the lines. The birth of the child is registered in the primary dentition, and perhaps the secondary first molars, as a broad, dark, hypomineralized line known as a neonatal line. It represents the change in the quality and quantity of the nutritional supply to the ameloblasts.

Bands of Hunter-Schreger

In a longitudinal ground section viewed with oblique, reflected light, broad alternating light and dark bands are seen. They extend through the inner two-thirds of the thickness of the enamel. This optical phenomenon is produced by light reflecting off groups of enamel rods as they weave from the dentinoenamel junction towards the surface. Those rods cut parallel to their long axis reflect large amounts of light and are seen as a bright band or parazone, whereas, those rods cut in a perpendicular plane reflect much less light and are seen as a darker band or diazone. This light and dark pattern is referred to as the bands of Hunter-Schreger (Figs. 2-8-1, 2).

Enamel Tufts

These structures originate at the dentinoenamel junction and extend outward to about one-fourth to one-third of the thickness of the enamel. They are composed of hypomineralized enamel rods, interrod enamel and organic matrix. They are oriented longitudinally along the length of the crown and are best seen in transverse ground sections. When a thick ground section is viewed under low magnification, they resemble a "tuft of grass" (Figs. 2-10-1, 2, 3). The winding, ribbon-like appearance of the tuft may be related to the horizontal weaving of the enamel rods near the dentinoenamel junction (Fig. 2- C: a, b).

Enamel Lamellae

The enamel lamellae are thin, ribbon-like hypomineralized structures that extend in from the enamel surface toward the dentinoenamel junction (Fig. 2-10-1). Some lamella may occasionally extend into the dentin. Lamella are arranged in a longitudinal and radial fashion from the tip of the crown to the cervical margin. They are best visualized in a transverse ground section of the cervical half of the crown. Those lamella formed during the formation of the crown are filled with organic material and cell debris, while those formed after eruption are filled by organic material derived from the saliva. These latter lamellae become more numerous with increasing age.

Enamel Spindles

The terminal ends of some dentinal tubules extend across the dentinoenamel junction and into enamel for a short distance. They are seen as small, dark, irregular or spiral-shaped structures. Each represents an odontoblast process that extended between the immature ameloblasts before the initiation of enamel formation and remained there until after enamel was formed (Fig. 2-G, Figs. 2-11-1, 2). They are normally filled with dentinal fluid. Their dark appearance is due to the presence of air and debris resulting from the preparation of the section. They occur most often along the dentinoenamel junction under the cusp tip or incisal edge where the junction is sharply bent. In most cases, they are not aligned along the same path as the enamel rods.

Dentinoenamel Junction

The dentinoenamel junction is a scalloped interface between enamel and dentin with numerous convexities facing the dentin (Fig. 2-G; Fig. 2-12-1). The close relationship between the dentin and the enamel rods can be seen in scanning electron micrographs (Fig. 2-12-2). If the enamel is removed, the surface of the dentin appears to be composed of pits or depressions (Fig. 2-8-2, Figs. 2-12-1, 2; Figs. 2-13-1, 2). This appearance is more evident in the mid-coronal region. Near the cervical margin, the dentinoenamel junction is smoother. This inter-digitation between enamel and dentin increases the surface area and mechanical strength of the junction.

Even though nerve endings have not been in enamel nor within dentin further than about 200 μm from the pulpal-dentin border, discomfort is often experienced when a bur passes through the dentinoenamel junction. According to the hydrodynamic theory of pain transmission, the movement of the dentinal fluid from the spindle into dentin is detected by the pulpal nerve endings and perceived as pain.

Perikymata

The enamel surface of a tooth that has received minimal abrasion presents several features. Aside from the longitudinal lamellae and cracks, there are shallow horizontal grooves or furrows called perikymata. These grooves represent the lines of Retzius as they meet the surface of the enamel. The perikymata are closely spaced near the cervical margin, become further apart in the mid-coronal region, and are absent at the cusp tips and incisal edges.

The tooth can be divided into the crown and the root. The anatomic crown is covered by enamel and the anatomic root is covered by cementum. Both tissues are supported by dentin which comprises the bulk of the tooth. The enamel is thickest in the cusp tip and tapers to an edge at the cervical margin.

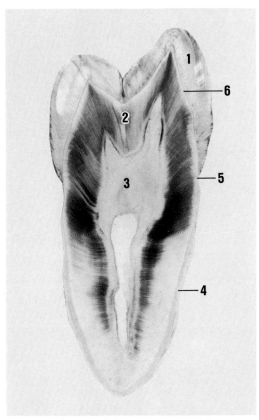

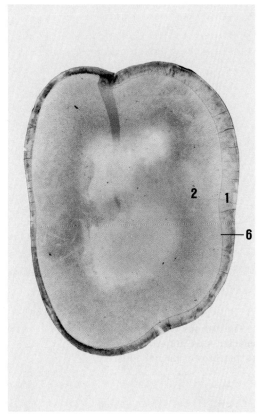

Fig. 2-1-1 Longitudinal mesial-distal ground section of the maxillary second premolar. X6

Fig. 2-1-2 Transverse section of the crown of the first maxillary molar. Ground section X6

---

1. Enamel
2. Dentin
3. Pulp cavity or chamber
4. Cementum
5. Cementoenamel junction
6. Dentinoenamel junction

Groups of enamel rods follow a wavy course from the dentinoenamel junction towards the surface of the tooth. In an oblique or transverse section, the enamel rods appear gnarled or twisted due to various orientations of the rods.

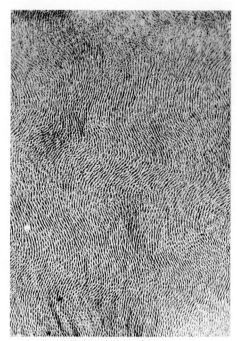

Fig. 2-2-1 Irregular orientation of enamel rods. Ground section X200

The various curvatures of the enamel rods are closely related to the brown enamel tufts.

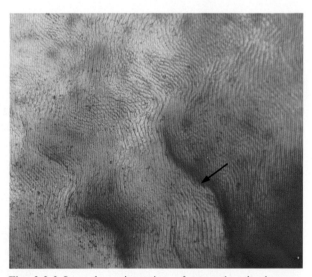

Fig. 2-2-2 Irregular orientation of enamel rods close to the dentinoenamel junction with enamel tufts (arrow). Ground section X350

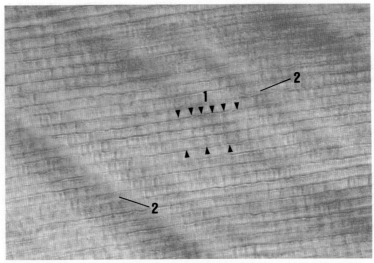

Fig. 2-3-1 Cross-striations are perpendicular to the long axis of the enamel rods. Several lines or striae of Retzius course obliquely across the enamel rods. Longitudinal ground section of enamel rods. Cross-striations and striae of Retzius are shown. Ground section X800

1. Cross-striation 2. Striae of Retzius

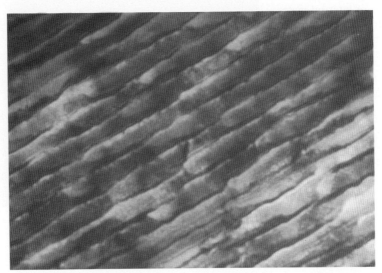

Fig. 2-3-2 Longitudinal ground section of enamel rods. The enamel rod is 4-6fm in width. X1,500

Enamel rods cut perpendicular to their long axis appear as arcades or keyholes.

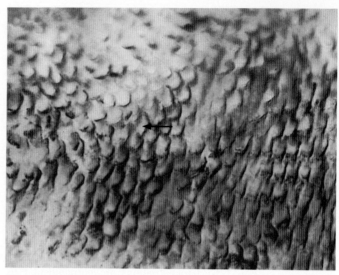

Fig. 2-4-1 Cross and oblique section of enamel rods. Ground section X1,200

The enamel rod sheath contains slightly more organic matrix than the enamel rod or interrod material. In this section, the organic matrix is intensely stained which outlines the enamel rod.

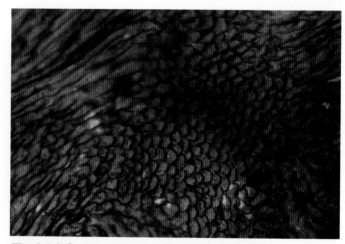

Fig. 2-4-2 Cross section of enamel rods. Ground section Carbol fuchsin stain X1,000

Arrow indicates the enamel rod (head).

The enamel rod is divided into 4-6 μm "blocks" or segments by cross-striations (dark bands).

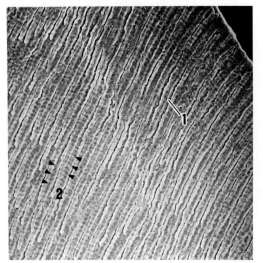

Fig. 2-5-1 Scanning electron micrograph of an etched, longitudinal ground section of enamel rods. Cross-striations of an enamel rod are indicated by arrowheads. X800

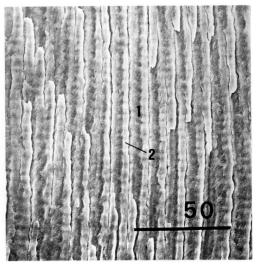

Fig. 2-5-2 Higher magnification of Fig. 3-5-1. X1,500

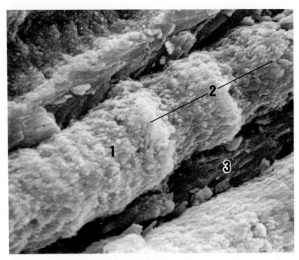

Fig. 2-5-3 Higher magnification of Fig. 3-5-1 showing cross-striations as varicosities. X7,000

The pattern of cross-striations denotes the daily apposition of enamel matrix. The expansions seen along the enamel rod may be produced by a slowing of the backward movement of the ameloblasts.

1. Enamel rod
2. Cross-striation

3. Interrod substance

In the mid-coronal region of the crown, the enamel rods appear as keyhole-shaped structures. Refer to Fig. 2-7-1.

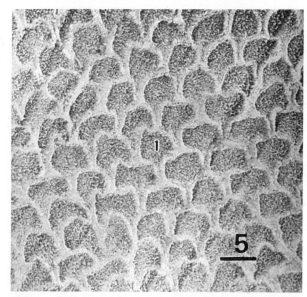

Fig. 2-6-1 Scanning electron micrograph of etched, transverse sectioned enamel rods. X3,500

Transversely-sectioned enamel rods are divided into two parts: head and tail. The tail is located between adjacent heads and corresponds to interrod enamel. The enamel rod sheath encloses the head and contains organic matrix and recrystallized hydroxyapatite crystals which are more acid-resistant. The rod sheath appears as a ridge.

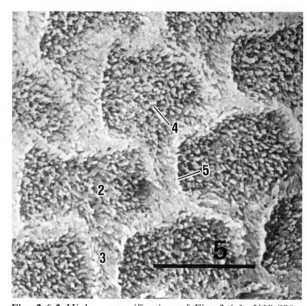

Fig. 2-6-2 Higher magnification of Fig. 3-6-1. X10,000

1. Enamel rod
2. Enamel rod head
3. Enamel rod tail
4. Enamel hydroxyapatite crystal
5. Enamel rod sheath

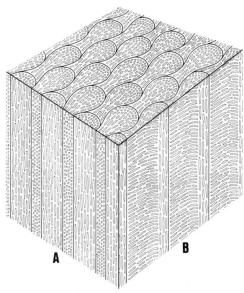

Fig. 2-7-1 The orientation of the hydroxyapatite crystals varies according to the plane of section and the location within the enamel rod. This shows the crystal orientation within a block of enamel cut in three planes each perpendicular to the other.

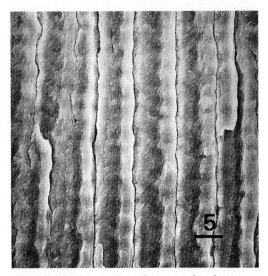

Fig. 2-7-2 In this section, the enamel rods are cut parallel to their long axis. The crystals in the head (right side) are cut lengthwise, while those in the tail (left side) are cut obliquely. Scanning electron micrograph of etched longitudinally sectioned enamel rods as they would appear in the **B** Face of Fig. 2-7-1. X2,000

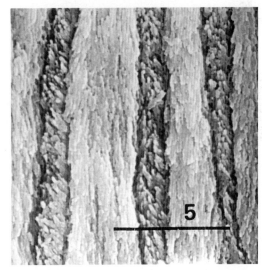

Fig. 2-7-3 In this section, the enamel rods are cut perpendicular to their long axis. The crystals in the head are cut lengthwise, while those in the tail are cut transversely. Scanning electron micrograph of etched longitudinally sectioned enamel rods as they would appear in the **A** Face of Fig. 2-7-1. X4,000

A longitudinally cut ground section of a tooth illuminated by reflected oblique light will show light and dark bands. The dark bands or diazones extend about two-thirds of the distance from the dentinoenamel junction to the surface of the tooth. The rods within the diazone are cut perpendicular to their long axis. In the light bands or parazones, the enamel rods are cut parallel to their long axis. Since the enamel rods in the outer one-third course straight to the surface, this region also appears light.

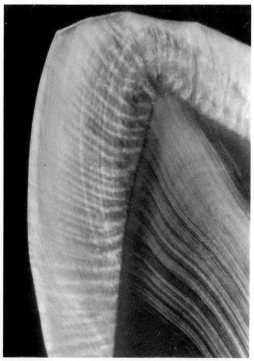

Fig. 2-8-1 Microphotograph of a longitudinal ground section viewed by reflected light demonstrating the bands of Hunter-Schreger. X15

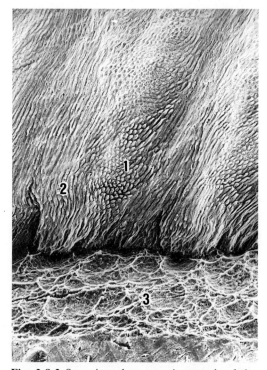

Fig. 2-8-2 Scanning electron micrograph of the dentinoenamel junction showing the pattern of the enamel rods that are seen as the bands of Hunter-Schreger. X200

1. Diazone 2. Parazone 3. Dentinoenamel junction

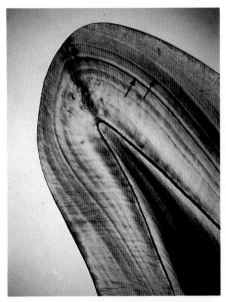

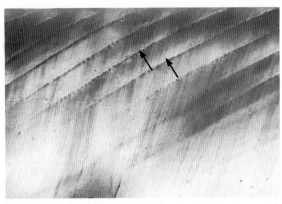

Fig. 2-9-2 Microphotograph of a longitudinal ground section demonstrating the striae of Retzius. X1,000

Fig. 2-9-1 The lines or striae of Retzius at the incisal edge do not reach the surface but arch over the tip of the dentinoenamel junction. Microphotograph of an incisal edge of a longitudinal ground section showing the striae of Retzius. X20

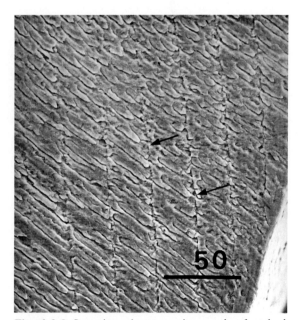

Fig. 2-9-3 Scanning electron micrograph of etched enamel showing the striae of Retzius. X500

Arrow indicates a striae of Retzius.

Enamel tufts originate at the dentinoenamel junction and extend into the enamel for about one-third of it's thickness. Their distribution is somewhat regular around the junction. Enamel lamellae extend from the surface of the tooth and may reach into the dentin. They are randomly distributed and are usually filled with organic material from the saliva.

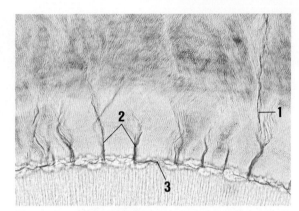

Fig. 2-10-1 Microphotograph of a transverse ground section along the dentinoenamel junction demonstrating enamel tufts and enamel lamella. X100

Enamel tufts are composed of hypomineralized rods, interrod material and organic matrix.

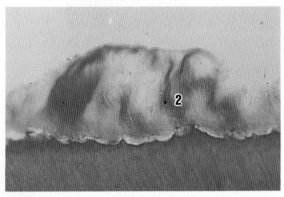

Fig. 2-10-2 Microphotograph of a partially demineralized transverse ground section showing enamel tufts. H-E stain X100

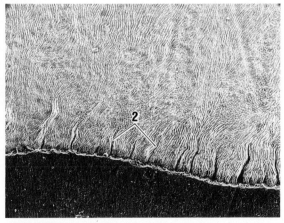

Fig. 2-10-3 Scanning electron micrograph of an etched transverse ground section showing enamel tufts. X100

1. Enamel lamella
2. Enamel tufts
3. Dentinoenamel junction

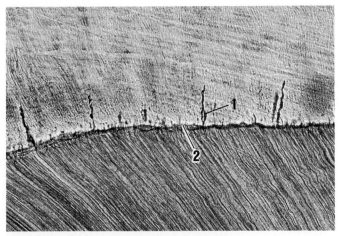

Some of the dentinal tubules extend for a short distance into the enamel. These terminal endings are seen as dilated, twisted structures called enamel spindles. They are usually filled with air from processing and appear dark.

Fig. 2-11-1 Microphotograph of a transverse ground section along the dentinoenamel junction. The enamel spindle is oriented obliquely to the dentinal tubules. X100

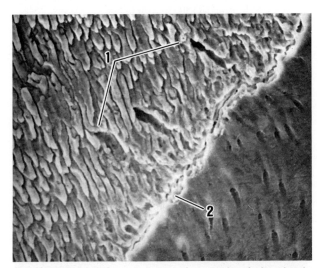

Fig. 2-11-2 Scanning electron micrograph of the dentinoenamel junction that shows enamel spindles as cavities among the enamel rods. The enamel spindles are not aligned with the enamel rods. X400

---

1. Enamel spindle

2. Dentinoenamel junction

The dentinoenamel junction is an irregular scalloped border. Depressions or bays are evident within the dentin surface.

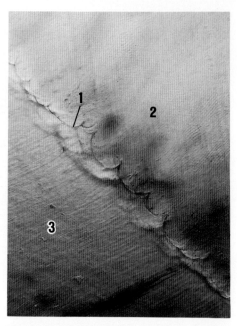

Fig. 2-12-1 Microphotograph of a longitudinal ground section that demonstrates the scalloped nature of the dentinoenamel junction. X150

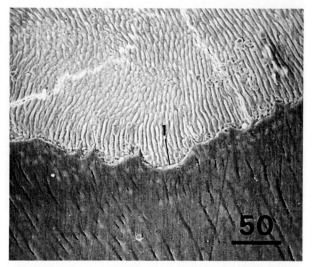

Fig. 2-12-2 Scanning electron micrograph of the dentinoenamel junction. X150

1. Dentinoenamel junction
2. Enamel

3. Dentin

The surface of the dentin displays a number of irregular depressions of varying sizes. The enamel was removed by decalcification.

The dentinoenamel junction near the cervical margin is relatively smooth.

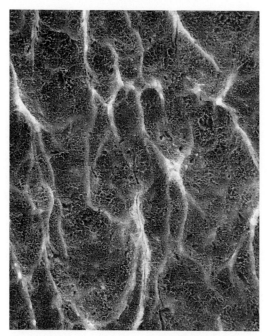

Fig. 2-13-1 Scanning electron micrograph of the surface of dentin showing the variable nature of the dentinoenamel junction. X500

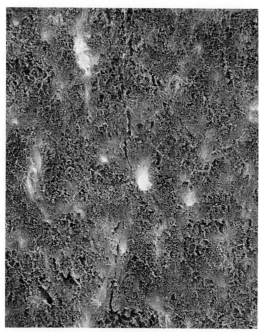

Fig. 2-13-2 Scanning electron micrograph of the dentinoenamel junction. X500

3

Tooth Structure:
Dentin

Tooth Structure: Dentin

The formation of dentin is a function of the cells of the dental papilla, which are of ectomesenchymal origin. Dentin is produced by peripheral cells of the dental papilla called odontoblasts. Dentin formation begins in the cusp tip or incisal edge region and continues apically until the anatomic root is completed. This site of deposition will mark the position of the dentinoenamel junction. Dentin formation occurs prior to and is essential for the formation of enamel. The dental papilla will remain as the dental pulp within the central region of the tooth after the tooth is completely formed.

Dentin forms the major bulk of the tooth. Coronal dentin supports the enamel of the crown and radicular dentin forms the roots and is covered by cementum. The inorganic content, about 70%, is in the form of hydroxyapatite. Therefore, the hardness of dentin is appreciably less than that of enamel. However, dentin is harder than bone and cementum and is more elastic than enamel. The organic matrix is composed mainly of collagen fibrils and ground substance (Figs. 3-5-1, 2; Fig. 3-6-2).

Dentin is produced by odontoblasts at a rate of about 4 μm/day. This daily deposition is marked by faint imbrication lines of von Ebner. These lines correspond to the enamel rod cross-striations. The more broadly spaced contour lines of Owen match the striae of Retzius. These contour lines indicate the appositional pattern or the location of the pulpal surface of the dentin at successive stages in the formation of the dentin. Once initiated, the formation of dentin will continue throughout the life of a tooth resulting in the gradual reduction in the size of the pulp chamber.

Dentinal Tubules

As the main body of the odontoblast retreats from the dentinoenamel junctions during dentin formation, it leaves behind a cytoplasmic extension or process (Tomes' dentinal fiber) that elongates with continued deposition of dentin. This process becomes enclosed by dentin, thus lying within a tubule (Figs. 3-3-1, 2; 3-4-1, 2; Figs. 3-6-1, 2; Figs. 3-7-1, 2). The region of dentin near the dentinoenamel junction has numerous tubules, some of which pass into enamel as enamel spindles (Fig. 3-1-1). Most of these tubules have many fine lateral branches less than 1 μm in diameter. These branches anastomose with others within this region to form an extensive network (Figs. 3-1-1, 2; Figs 3-2-1, 2). The dentin found between the dentinal tubules is called intertubular dentin. Each odontoblast process within it's tubule becomes surrounded by a layer of peritubular dentin. This highly mineralized, collagen-poor peritubular matrix is deposited on the inner wall of the dentinal tubules. This layer is lost during decalcification procedures (Figs. 3-8-1, 2; Figs. 3-9-1, 2).

Dentin Formation and Mineralization

The odontoblasts deposit dentin matrix as a nonmineralized material called predentin. After a period of time, crystals of hydroxyapatite appear within the matrix to form mineralized dentin. The pattern of mineralization takes two different forms: globular and linear. Globular mineralization develops as concentric circles around a central point to form a sphere or calcoglobule. Following the fusion of several mineralized globules, a broad surface of mineralization is formed which is described as linear mineralization (Fig. 3-A; Figs. 3-13-1, 2; Fig. 3-14-1).

Interglobular Dentin

The term, interglobular dentin, refers to an area found between globules of mineralization that failed to mineralize completely. This type of hypomineralized dentin is usually found some distance from the dentinoenamel junction (Figs.

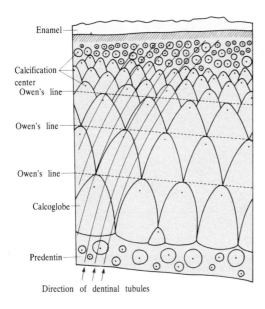

Fig. 3-A Diagram illustrates the change from globular to linear patterns of mineralization in dentin.

3-13-1, 2; Fig. 3-14-1; Figs. 3-15-1, 2; Fig. 3-16-1; Figs. 3-17-1, 2). In certain H-E stained sections, a pattern of nonmineralized regions may be seen as an interglobular net (Figs. 3-18-1, 2).

Granular Layer of Tomes

In ground sections, a narrow band of dentin located immediately beneath the dentinocemental junction has a granular appearance. This granular layer of Tomes represents fluid-filled spaces formed by the terminal expansion or dilation of dentinal tubules (Fig. 3-19-2, Figs. 3-20-1, 2). The region between this granular layer and the dentinocemental junction is often referred to as intermediate cementum (Fig. 3-19-1).

Sclerotic Dentin and Dead Tracts

In some ground sections, especially of teeth from aged people, there are areas within the dentin that are translucent or transparent. This is due to the occlusion of the tubules over large areas by deposits of hydroxyapatite (Fig. 3-25-2; Figs. 3-26-1, 2; Figs. 3-27-1, 2). This translucent or sclerotic dentin is often seen in areas of low-grade, long-term stimulation, as in occlusal abrasion of cusp tips. In some sections, the dentinal tubules appear dark or empty with the pulpal-dentin ends sealed by dentin (Fig. 3-25-1). Such appearance is often associated with a more rapid, acute stimulation. A group of these dark tubules have been referred to as "dead tracts."

The dentin that is formed prior to the completion of the anatomic root is called primary dentin, that formed afterwards is secondary dentin. Primary dentin can also be divided into mantle dentin which is the first-formed 20-30 μm layer and circumpulpal dentin. The change from primary to secondary dentin is marked by an abrupt change in the pattern of the dentinal tubules or Schreger's line (Figs. 3-21-1, 2, 3). The rate of secondary dentin formation is very slow, perhaps less than 1 μm/day. In response to a noxious stimulus, reparative or tertiary dentin may be rapidly formed (Fig. 3-21-1; Figs. 3-23-1, 2; Figs. 3-24-1, 2; Fig. 3-25-1). This type of dentin is characterized by having very few, irregularly-arranged tubules in a low-mineralized matrix. If the rate of formation is very rapid, the matrix-forming cells may become buried. This dentin may be referred to as osteodentin.

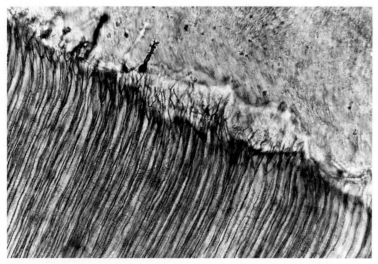

Fig. 3-1-1 Dentinal tubules along the scalloped dentinoenamel junction. Ground section. X150

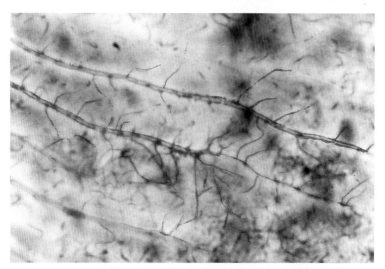

Fig. 3-1-2 Dentinal tubules illustrating lateral branching. Ground section. X920

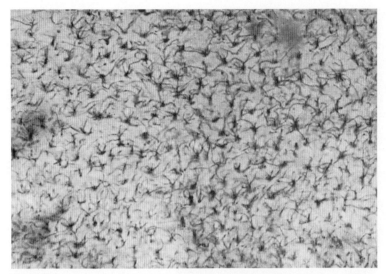

Fig. 3-2-1 Dentinal tubules in a transverse demineralized section. Silver impregnation X300

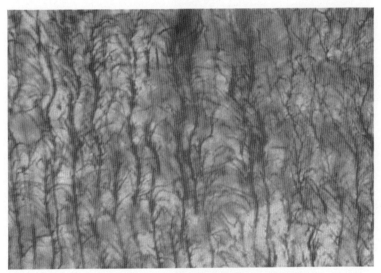

Fig. 3-2-2 Dentinal tubules in longitudinal demineralized section showing extensive branching. Silver impregnation X300

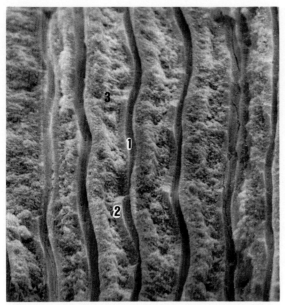

Fig. 3-3-1 Scanning electron micrograph of dentinal tubules in longitudinal section. X2,650

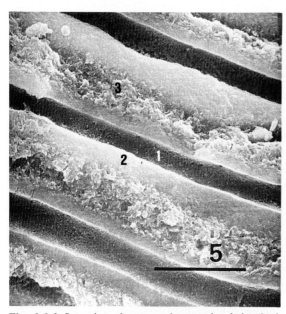

Fig. 3-3-2 Scanning electron micrograph of dentinal tubules at a greater magnification. A comparison of peritubular and intertubular dentin is shown. X3,390

1. Dentinal tubules
2. Peritubular dentin
3. Intertubular dentin

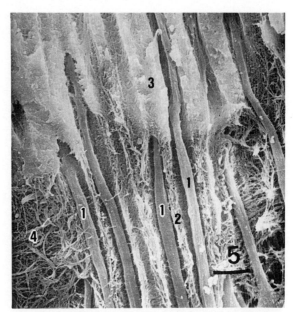

Fig. 3-4-1 Scanning electron micrograph of longitudinal sectioned dentinal tubules containing odontoblast processes. X2,700

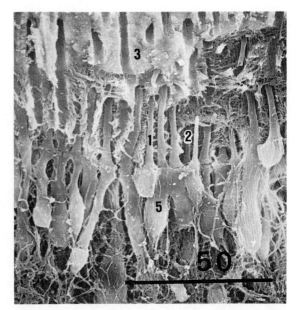

Fig. 3-4-2 Scanning electron micrograph of odontoblasts along the pulpal-dentin border. X2,650

1. Odontoblast process
2. Predentin
3. Dentin

4. Matrix collagen fibers
5. Odontoblast

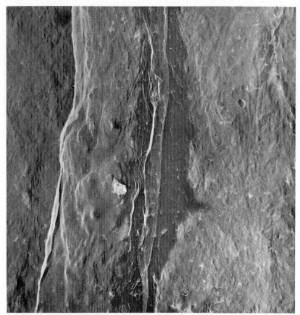

Fig. 3-5-1 Scanning electron micrograph of a replica illustrating dentinal tubules. X8,745

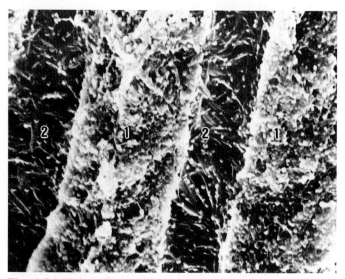

Fig. 3-5-2 Enlarged scanning electron micrograph of dentinal tubules. X13,000
1. Dentin matrix   2. Dentinal tubule

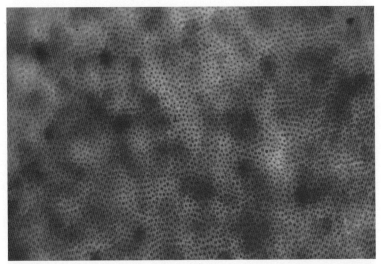

Fig. 3-6-1 Dentinal tubules in transverse section. Silver impregnation X200

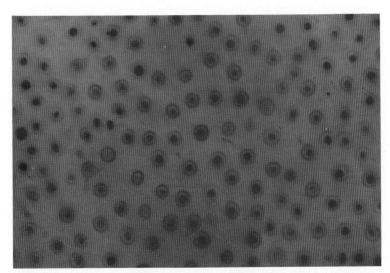

Fig. 3-6-2 Higher magnification of Fig. 3-6-1 of dentinal tubules in transverse section. Silver impregnation X1,000

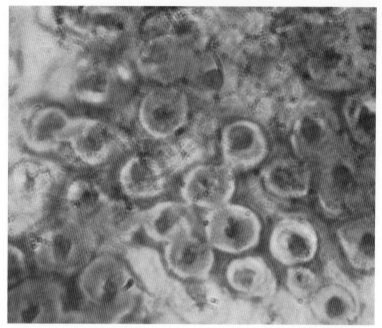

Fig. 3-7-1 Dentinal tubules in transverse section. Silver impregnation X2,200

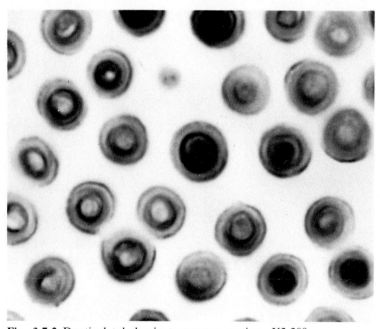

Fig. 3-7-2 Dentinal tubules in transverse section. X2,200

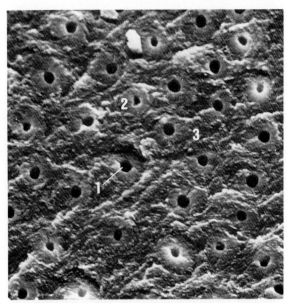

Fig. 3-8-1 Scanning electron micrograph of dentin and dentinal tubules in transverse section. X1,924

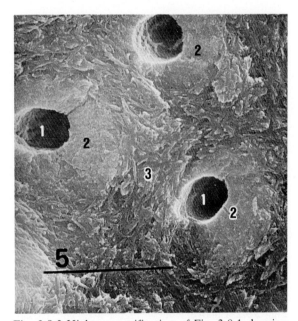

Fig. 3-8-2 Higher magnification of Fig. 3-8-1 showing dentinal tubules in transverse section with peritubular dentin. X8,000

1. Dentinal tubules
2. Peritubular dentin

3. Intertubular dentin

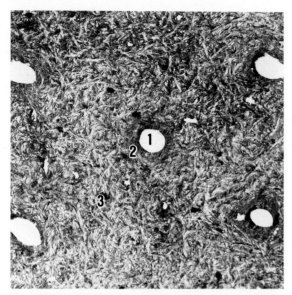

Fig. 3-9-1 Transmission electron micrograph of dentin showing the collagenous fibrils of the dentin matrix around transverse sectioned dentinal tubules. X3,200

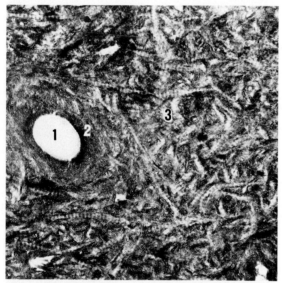

Fig. 3-9-2 Enlargement of Fig. 3-9-1. The typical cross-banding of collagen fibrils is seen in the matrix of intertubular dentin. The fibrous matrix of peritubular dentin does not contain cross-banded fibrils. Transmission electron micrograph. X8,000

1.	Dentinal tubules	**3.**	Intertubular dentin
2.	Peritubular dentin		

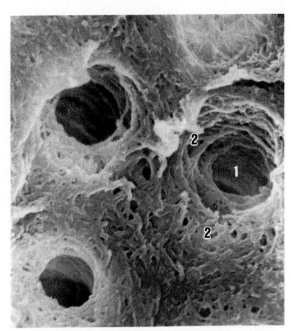

Fig. 3-10-1 Scanning electron micrograph of dentinal tubules in transverse section. X10,000

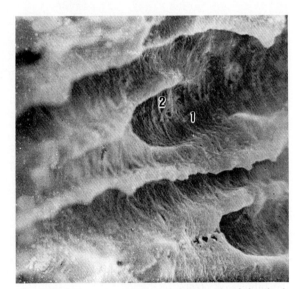

Fig. 3-10-2 Scanning electron micrograph of dentinal tubules in oblique section. X10,000

1. Dentinal tubules   2. Matrix fibers

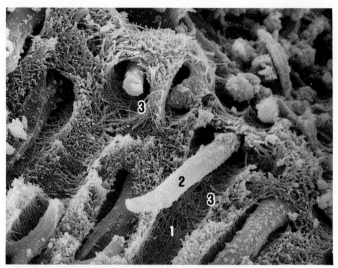

Fig. 3-11-1 Scanning electron micrograph of dentinal tubules within predentin in oblique section. The odontoblast process is seen within the tubule. X5,000

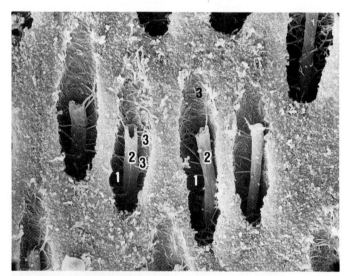

Fig. 3-11-2 Scanning electron micrograph of dentinal tubules in oblique section. Odontoblast processes are evident within the tubules. X5,000

1. Dentinal tubules   3. Matrix fibers
2. Odontoblast process

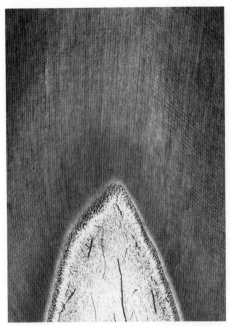

Fig. 3-12-1 Lines of von Ebner illustrating the daily increment of dentin formation. Demineralized section. H-E stain X80

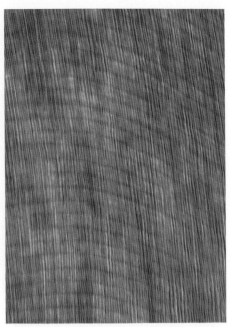

Fig. 3-12-2 Enlargement of Fig. 3-12-1 showing incremental lines of von Ebner. Demineralized section. H-E stain X300

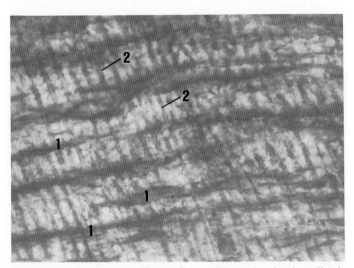

Fig. 3-12-3 Incremental lines of von Ebner in demineralized dentin. Silver impregnation X400
1. Incremental lines 2. Dentinal tubules

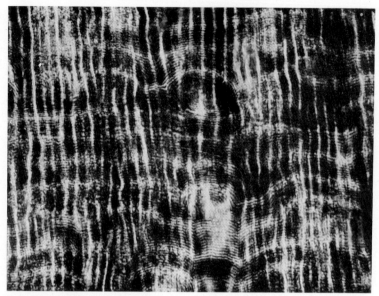

Fig. 3-13-1 Mixture of globular and linear patterns of mineralization. The calcoglobule contour can be seen. Silver impregnation X500 (Fujita T: Dental Histology, Ishiyaku, 1957)

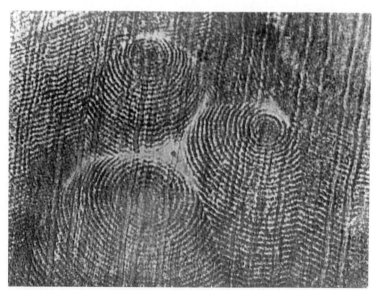

Fig. 3-13-2 The small angular region between the globules of dentin represents interglobular dentin. Silver impregnation X510 (Matsui T: Oral Histology, Tooth section, Nagasue, 1965)

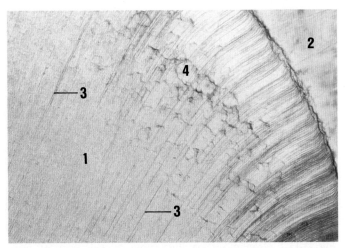

Fig. 3-14-1 Longitudinal ground section illustrating interglobular dentin. Silver impregnation (green filter) X36

The region of dentin between the dentinoenamel junction and the interglobular dentin has been referred to as mantle dentin. All dentin formed subsequent to mantle dentin is referred to as circumpulpal dentin.

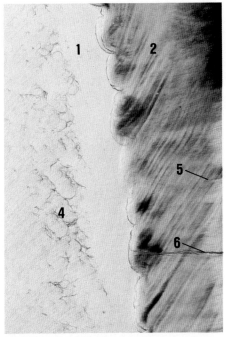

Fig. 3-14-2 Longitudinal ground section showing the scalloped nature of the dentinoenamel junction. Silver impregnation X72

1. Dentin
2. Enamel
3. Dentinal tubules
4. Interglobular dentin in circumpulpal dentin
5. Striae of Retzius
6. Enamel lamella

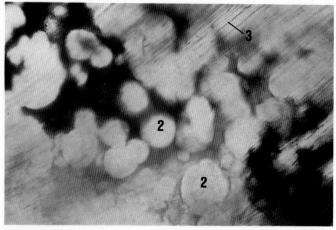

Fig. 3-15-1 Ground section illustrating calcoglobules of mineralized dentin and regions of hypomineralized interglobular dentin. Silver impregnation X200

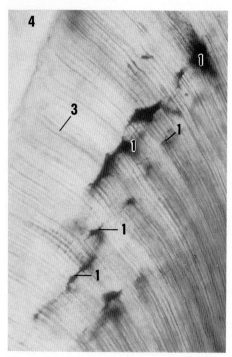

Multiple regions of interglobular dentin frequently follow a linear pattern and are found along the contour lines of Owen.

Fig. 3-15-2 Ground section of interglobular dentin aligned with a contour line of Owen. Silver impregnation X66

1.	Interglobular dentin	3.	Dentinal tubules
2.	Calcoglobules	4.	Enamel

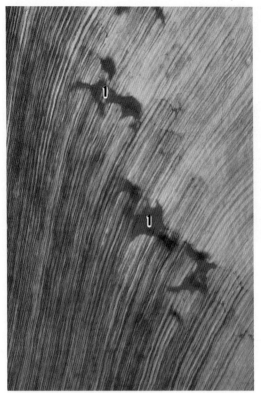

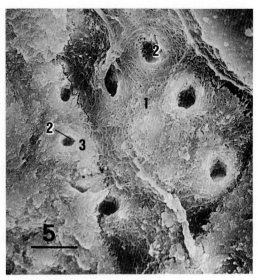

Fig. 3-16-2 Scanning electron micrograph of interglobular dentin and dentinal tubules in transverse section. X2,800

Fig. 3-16-1 Ground section of interglobular dentin. Silver impregnation-carbol fuchsin stain X66

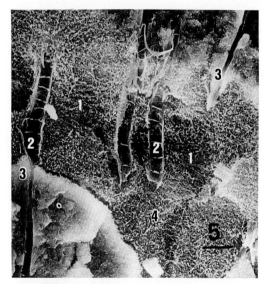

Fig. 3-16-3 Scanning electron micrograph of interglobular dentin and dentinal tubules in longitudinal section. X2,800

1. Interglobular dentin   3. Peritubular dentin
2. Dentinal tubules   4. Matrix fibers

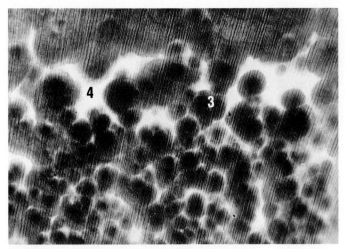

Fig. 3-17-1 Longitudinal ground section of dentin. X100

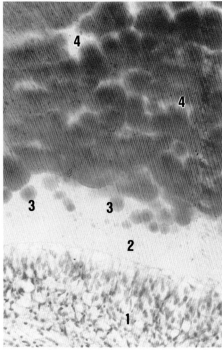

Fig. 3-17-2 Demineralized section of dentin. Compare with Fig. 3-17-1. Silver impregnation X100

---

1. Dental pulp
2. Predentin

3. Calcoglobules
4. Interglobular dentin

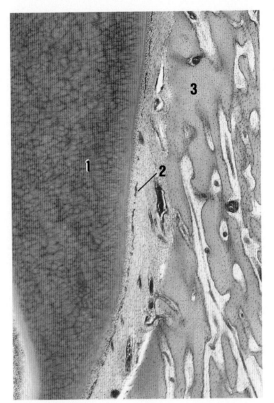

Fig. 3-18-1 Network pattern of interglobular dentin. Demineralized section H-E stain X40

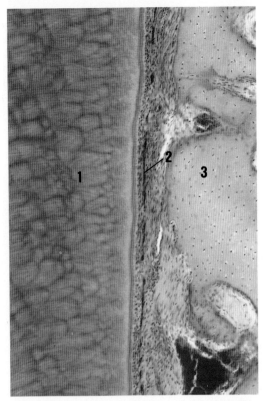

Fig. 3-18-2 Network pattern of interglobular dentin. Demineralized section H-E stain X100

1. Interglobular dentin network
2. Epithelial rest of Malassez
3. Alveolar bone

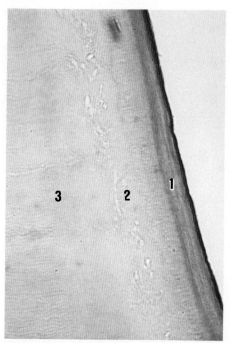

The region of the root just beneath the dentinocemental junction stains similar to that of dentin. This homogenous layer may be formed by the cells of Hertwig's epithelial root sheath. The region is referred to as intermediate cementum.

Fig. 3-19-1 Demineralized section showing intermediate cementum in the root. H-E stain X40

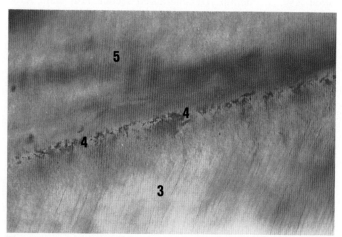

A granular layer can be seen beneath the dentinoenamel junction in this malformed tooth. This is not seen in a normal tooth. This layer may be due to odontoblasts becoming embedded during initial dentin formation. The origin of this layer is different from the granular layer of Tomes found in the root.

Fig. 3-19-2 Granular layer beneath the dentinoenamel junction. Silver impregnation X40

1. Cementum
2. Intermediate cementum
3. Dentin
4. Granular layer
5. Enamel

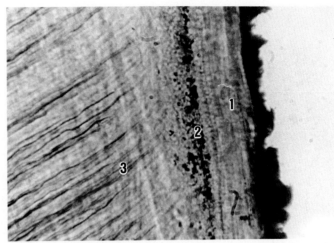

Fig. 3-20-1 Longitudinal ground section of the root showing the granular layer of Tomes. X200

Embedded cells within the granular layer of Tomes may originate from Hertwig's epithelial root sheath. The layer is composed principally of terminal dilations of dentinal tubules.

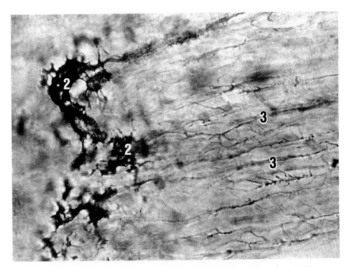

Fig. 3-20-2 Cell-like inclusions in the granular layer of Tomes. Ground section. X800

1. Cementum
2. Granular layer of Tomes
3. Dentinal tubules

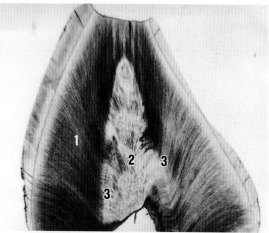

Fig. 3-21-1 Longitudinal ground section of a primary incisor. The change from primary to secondary dentin is marked by an abrupt change in tubular pattern. This line of directional change has been referred to as Schreger's line. X40

1. Primary dentin   2. Tertiary dentin   3. Schreger's line

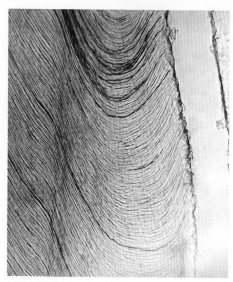

Fig. 3-21-2 Longitudinal ground section showing Schreger's line. X100

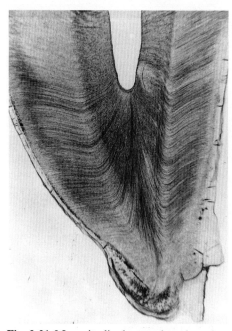

Fig. 3-21-3 Longitudinal ground section of a maxillary first premolar showing the change from primary to secondary dentin formation that corresponds to the completion of the anatomic root. X40

A large pulp stone or denticle has become attached to secondary dentin.

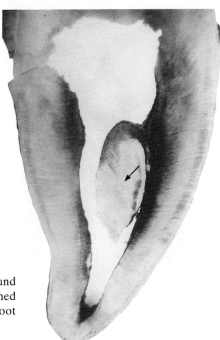

Fig. 3-22-1 Longitudinal ground section of a tooth root. Attached denticle (arrow) on wall of root canal. X35

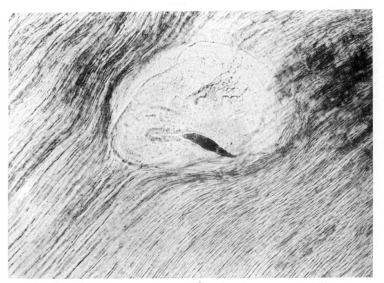

Fig. 3-22-2 Ground section of denticle embedded within dentin. X100

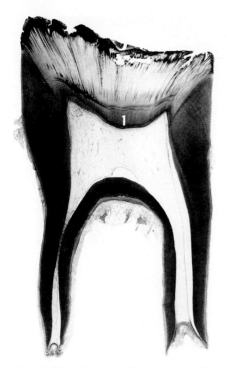

Fig. 3-23-1 Demineralized longitudinal
section of a molar tooth. X6

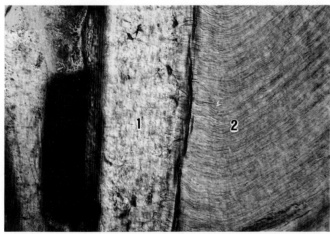

Fig. 3-23-2 Ground section of tooth showing primary dentin,
secondary dentin and tertiary or reparative dentin. X20

1. Tertiary or reparative dentin
2. Primary dentin (to the right of the number),
   secondary dentin (to the left)

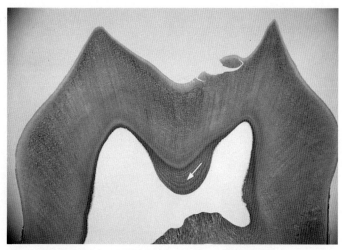

Fig. 3-24-1 Demineralized longitudinal section of a primary maxillary first molar. Reparative or tertiary dentin is seen on the roof of the pulp chamber (arrow) H-E stain. X10

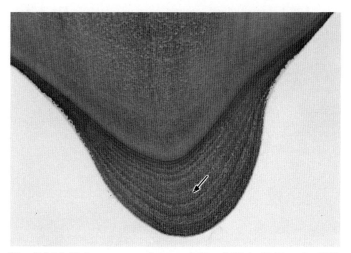

Fig. 3-24-2 Enlargement of part of Fig. 3-24-1. H-E stain X70

Arrow designates reparative or tertiary dentin

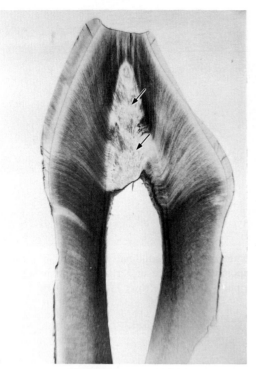 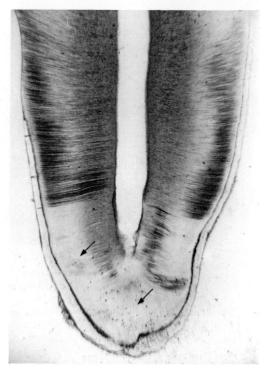

Fig. 3-25-1 Longitudinal ground section of a primary canine. X10 Arrows point to areas of reparative dentin.

Fig. 3-25-2 Longitudinal ground section of a root. X10 Arrows indicate areas of transparent dentin.

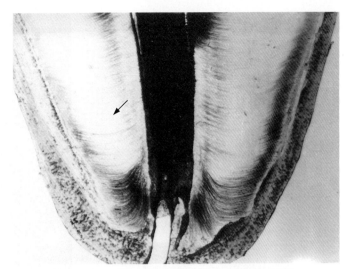

Fig. 3-26-1 Longitudinal ground section of root. X20

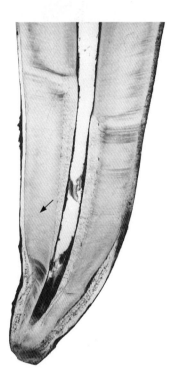

Fig. 3-26-2 Longitudinal ground section of root. X10

Arrow indicates transparent dentin.

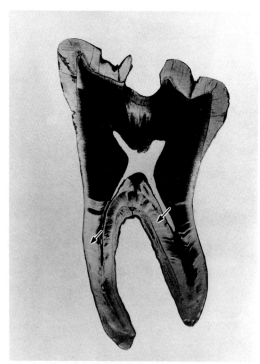

Fig. 3-27-1 Longitudinal ground section of a molar tooth. Transparent dentin appears as light areas of dentin. X4.4

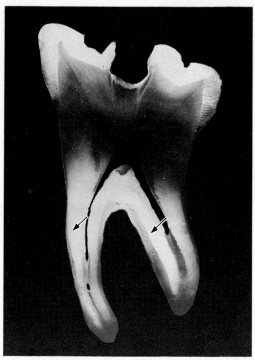

Fig. 3-27-2 Radiograph of the same tooth in Fig. 3-27-1. Areas of transparent dentin appear more radiopaque than regions of normal dentin. X4.4

Arrow designates transparent dentin.

It has been reported that sensory nerve fibers are present in every tenth dentinal tubule. These nerve fibers do not extend further than 200 μm from the pulpal-dentin border.

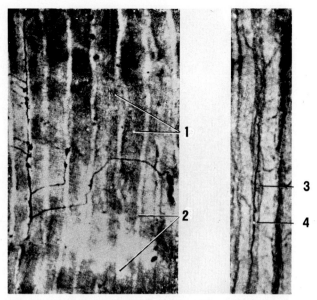

Fig. 3-28-1 Microphotograph of nerve fibers within dentin. Silver impregnation X1,000 (Tojoda, M., Dtsch Zahnaerztl Wochschr 37:641-5, 1934)

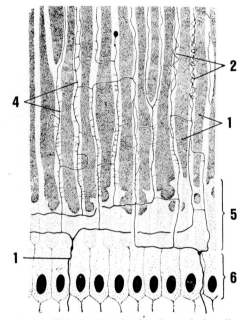

Fig. 3-28-2 Schematic drawing of the distribution of nerve fibers in dentin X1,200 (Tojoda, M., Dtsch Zahnaerztl Wochschr 37:641-5, 1934)

1. Dentin matrix
2. Dentinal tubules
3. Odontoblast process

4. Nerve fiber
5. Predentin
6. Odontoblast

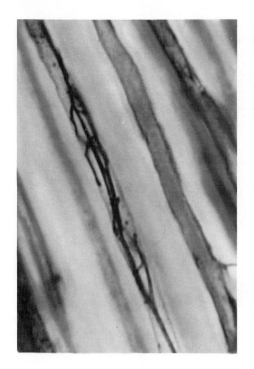

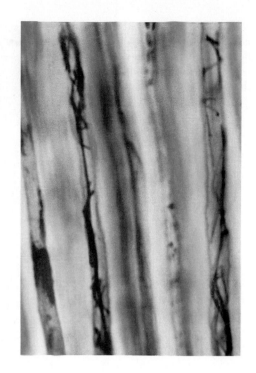

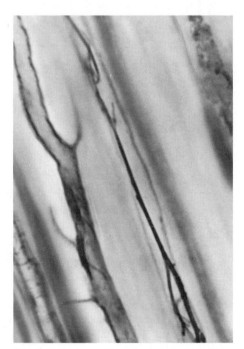

Fig. 3-29-1 Nerve fibers in dentinal tubules.
X1,900

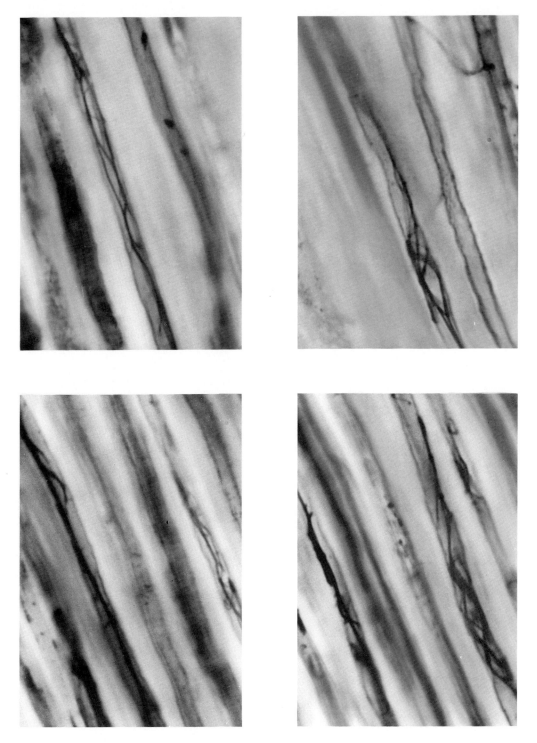

Fig. 3-29-2 Nerve fibers in dentinal tubules. X1,900

4

Dental Pulp

DENTAL PULP

The dental pulp arises from the ectomesenchyme of the dental papilla. The dental papilla is a highly vascular condensation of undifferentiated mesenchymal cells (Figs. 1-15-1, 2). These primitive cells will differentiate into odontoblasts, fibroblasts and other cells of the pulp. The fibroblasts will produce the fibers and ground substance of the pulp. The dental papilla serves to initiate the formation of enamel, produce the dentin of the tooth and remain as the connective tissue of the dental pulp. This specialized connective tissue contains all the cells and fibers of loose connective tissue with the exception of adipocytes and free elastic fibers (Fig. 4-2-1, 2). Elastic fibers are found only in the walls of the blood vessels.

The dental pulp passes through several stages before it reaches a mature state. After the deposition of the first layer of predentin, the dental papilla is referred to as the primitive or formative pulp. The formative pulp produces primary, and if necessary, reparative dentin, until the apices of the anatomic root(s) are completely formed. After the establishment of the fully-formed root, the dental pulp is described as being mature and produces secondary dentin. The mature pulp supplies nutrients to the odontogenic cells, contains sensory mechanisms for defense and produces secondary and reparative dentin. The dental pulp contains numerous blood vessels and nerves (Fig. 4-2-1, Figs. 4-3-3, 4,; Fig. 4-5-1, Fig. 4-6-1, Figs. 4-7-1, 2, 3; Fig. 4-9-2). Numerous lymphatic vessels are also found.

Pulp Cells

The most numerous pulp cells are the fibroblast. They are spindle or stellate-shaped with oval nuclei (Fig. 4-4-1, Fig. 4-6-2, Fig. 4-7-3, Fig. 4-11-1). They have elongated processes that may be linked by nexus to other fibroblasts (Figs. 4-3-1, 2; Fig. 4-4-1, Figs. 4-12-1 to 4-13-2). The fibroblasts are responsible for the production of both collagen and reticular fibers and the ground substance of the pulp. These cells may also function in the degradation of collagen. During the formation of mantle dentin, there appears among the odontoblast, large coiled, argyrophilic fibers called Korff's fibers (Fig. 4-4-2). They may be an artifact of staining. During circumpulpal dentin formation, their appearance decreases considerably. The arrangement of the cells within the pulp core is uniform except for two zones, the cell-rich and cell-free zones. The cell-rich zone is found in the outer region or parietal layer of the pulp core. It contains numerous fibroblasts and undifferentiated cells. It may represent a population of reserve cells. The cell-free zone of Weil is occasionally found between the cell-rich layer and the odontoblasts. It is best seen during the formation of secondary dentin. It is rarely seen during rapid dentin formation. This region consists of a fine network of collgenous and reticular fibers for the support of the fine nonmyelinated nerve fibers and small capillaries.

Besides odontoblasts and fibroblasts, other cells are found within the pulp core. These consists of macrophages or histiocytes, undifferentiated cells and an occasional mast cell. Defensive cells may also seen during periods of inflammation and include lymphocytes, plasma cells, neutrophils and eosinophils.

Odontoblasts

The odontoblasts arise from ectomesenchyme and produce the dentin matrix. These tall columnar cells are found lining the surface of the dental pulp (Figs. 4-1-1, 2; Figs. 4-2-1, 2; Figs. 4-3-1, 2; Fig. 4-4-1). The odontoblast is about 25 μm in height and 3-4 μm in width. It is cylindrical and longer in the coronal pulp, and more cuboidal in the middle of the root. It has a large oval nucleus positioned at the basal end of the cell with a cytoplasmic process extending from the distal end into a tubule in the dentin. This process has been termed Tomes' dentinal process or fiber. Controversy still exists as to how close the processes come to the dentinoenamel junction. The rate of dentin production may vary from more than 6-8 μm/day as in reparative dentin to much less than 1 μm/day in secondary dentin.

Blood Vessels and Nerves

Blood vessels are associated with the dental papilla during the early stages of tooth development. Proliferation of capillaries occurs with the initiation of dentin formation and, in addition, they appear among the folds of the outer enamel epithelium with the beginning of enamel formation.

In a fully-formed tooth, one or two arteries and one to three veins pass through the narrow apical foramina (Fig. 4-9-1, Fig. 4-14-1). The artery branches into arterioles that course longitudinally through the radicular pulp giving off an occasional branch (Fig. 4-5-1, Fig. 4-10-2). Extensive branching occurs in the coronal pulp. These smaller arterioles extend toward the odontoblasts and form into a rich subodontoblastic capillary plexus. From this plexus, small capillary loops may extend among the odontoblasts. The wall of the pulpal arteriole is much thinner in comparison to arterioles in the rest of the body.

Nerves become associated with the developing tooth during the apposition stage of dentin and enamel. In the mature tooth, two types of nerves are found in the pulp: coarse myelinated (sensory) and nonmyelinated (vasomotor) (Fig. 4-8-2, Fig. 4-11-2). Nerves enter the apical foramen and coarse with the large blood vessels. In the coronal pulp, smaller branches extend to the cell-rich zone where the myelinated nerves form the parietal plexus of Rashkow. Fine nerves fibers extend from this plexus toward the predentin, losing their myelin sheath and pass among the odontoblasts. Some of these fibers continue into the dentinal tubules along with the odontoblast processes. About every one in ten tubules may contain a nerve fiber. Controversy also exists as to how close the nerve fibers extend toward the dentinoenamel junction. Stimulation of these nerves is perceived only as pain. The nonmyelinated nerves coarse with the blood vessels. Stimulation of these nerves results in increased dentin formation.

Age Changes in the Pulp

The dimensions of the pulp chamber decreases with increasing age of the tooth. The fibrous component increases in density as the cellular population, vascularity and innervation decreases. The frequency of intrapulpal calcifications also increases. These mineralized bodies are referred to as denticles or pulp stones (Fig. 4-10-1; Figs. 4-14-1, 2). True denticles, which are surrounded by odontoblasts, are found near the apical foramen, whereas the false denticles occur more frequently in the coronal pulp. More diffuse calcifications are found in the radicular pulp.

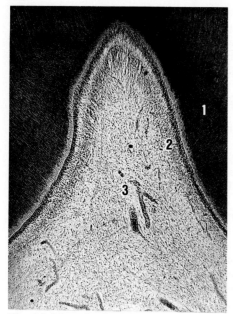

Fig. 4-1-1 Longitudinal section of the coronal pulp. H-E stain X20

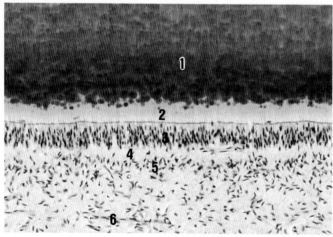

Fig. 4-1-2 Longitudinal section of the coronal pulp along the pulpal-dentin border. H-E stain X180

1. Dentin
2. Predentin
3. Odontoblastic layer

4. Cell-free zone of Weil
5. Cell-rich zone
6. Blood vessel

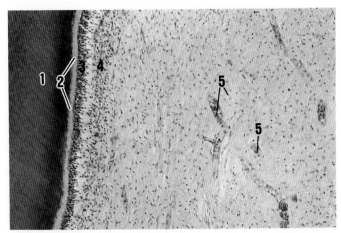

Fig. 4-2-1 Longitudinal section of the coronal pulp which shows the vascularity of the pulp core. H-E stain X80

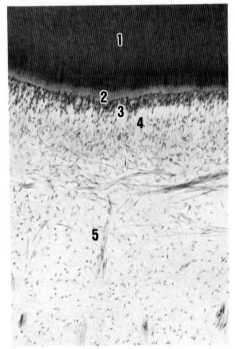

Fig. 4-2-2 Longitudinal section of the coronal pulp. H-E stain X150

1. Dentin
2. Predentin
3. Odontoblastic layer
4. Cell-rich zone
5. Blood vessel

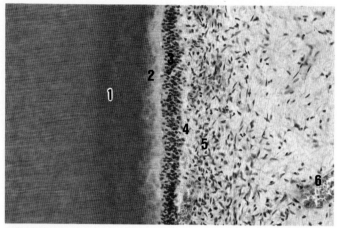

Fig. 4-3-1 Longitudinal section of the coronal pulp showing the dense cellular condensation along the pulpal-dentin border. H-E stain X180

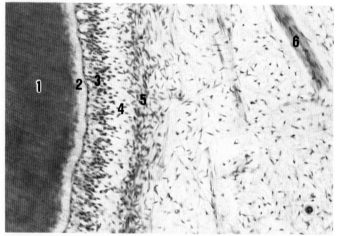

Fig. 4-3-2 This section of the coronal pulp shows the odontogenic zones of the pulp including the odontoblasts, the cell-free zone and the cell-rich zone. H-E stain X180

1.	Dentin	**4.**	Cell-free zone of Weil
2.	Predentin	**5.**	Cell-rich zone
3.	Odontoblastic layer	**6.**	Blood vessel

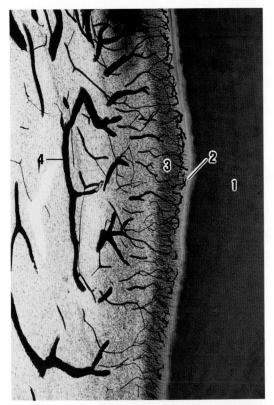

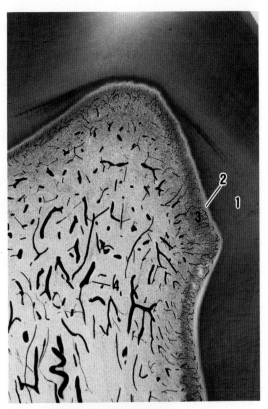

Fig. 4-3-3 Longitudinal section of the coronal pulp of a tooth from a dog that was vascularly instilled with India ink to illustrate the large blood vessels of the pulp core and the fine vascular plexus associated with the odontoblast layer. X60

Fig. 4-3-4 Longitudinal section of the coronal pulp similar to Fig. 4-3-3. X40

1. Dentin
2. Predentin

3. Odontoblastic layer
4. Blood vessel

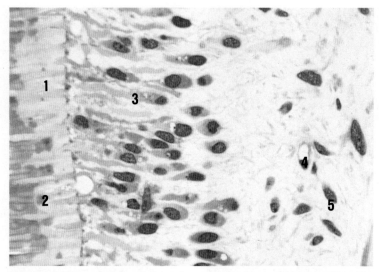

Fig. 4-4-1 Thin section of the odontoblastic layer. H-E stain X1,200
1. Predentin   2. Calcoglobules   3. Odontoblast   4. Capillary   5. Pulp cell

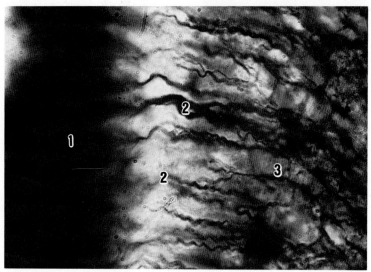

Fig. 4-4-2 Appearance of Korff's fibers seen during early dentin formation. Silver impregnation X1,200

1. Predentin   2. Korff's fibers   3. Odontoblastic layer

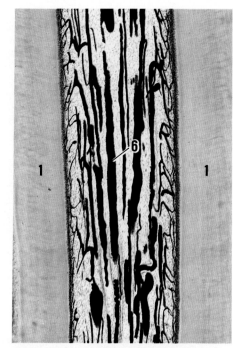

Fig. 4-5-1 Longitudinal section of the radicular pulp of a tooth from a dog that was vascular instilled with India ink to show the course of the major blood vessels within the pulp canal. H-E stain X20

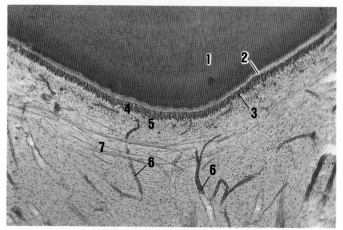

Fig. 4-5-2 Dental pulp along the surface of the dentin showing blood vessels and nerves. H-E stain X60

1.	Dentin	**5.**	Cell-rich zone
2.	Predentin	**6.**	Blood vessel
3.	Odontoblastic layer	**7.**	Nerve plexus of Raschkow
4.	Cell-free zone of Weil		

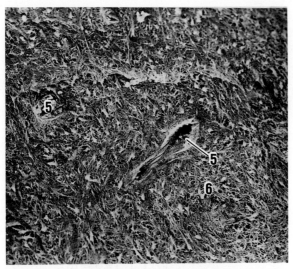

Fig. 4-6-1 Scanning electron micrograph of the core of the dental pulp. X400

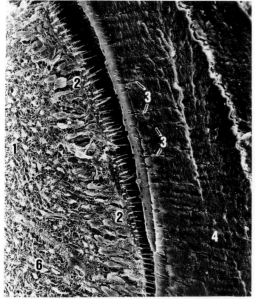

Fig. 4-6-2 Scanning electron micrograph of a longitudinal section along the pulpal-dentin border showing dentinal tubules and dentin matrix. X400

1. Dental pulp
2. Odontoblastic layer
3. Dentinal tubules
4. Dentin matrix
5. Blood vessel
6. Cells and fibers of the pulp

114

This special stain was used to illustrate the collagen fibers of the pulp which stain blue. Blood vessels, nerves and the cells of the pulp stain red.

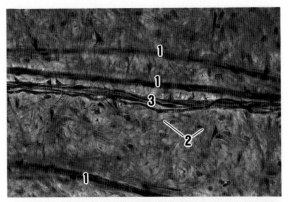

Fig. 4-7-1 Dental pulp. Azan stain X300

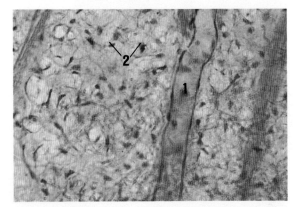

Fig. 4-7-2 Dental pulp. H-E stain X300

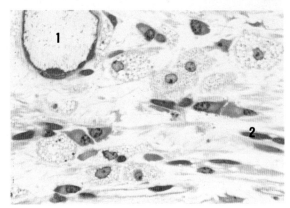

Fig. 4-7-3 Thin section of the dental pulp. Toluidine blue stain X1,200

1. Blood vessel
2. Pulp cell

3. Nerve fibers

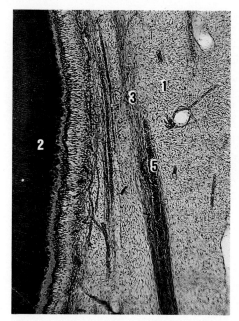

Fig. 4-8-1 Dental pulp. H-E stain X100

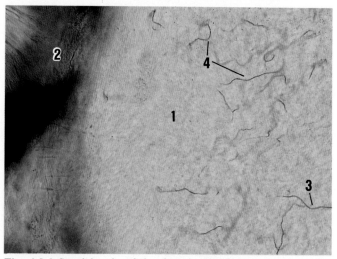

Fig. 4-8-2 Special stain of the dental pulp demonstrates myelinated nerves fibers. Silver impregnation X180

1. Dental pulp
2. Dentin
3. Nerve fiber bundles in the dental pulp
4. Nerve fibers
5. Blood vessel

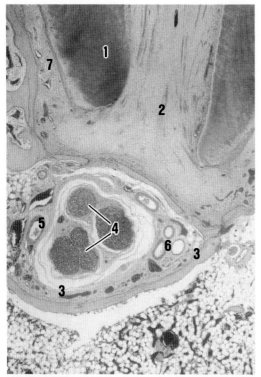

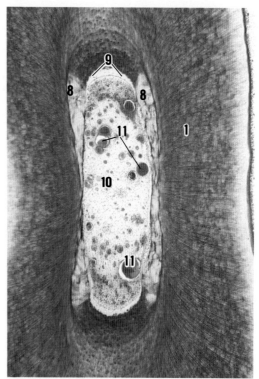

Fig. 4-9-1 The relationship of the apical foramen of an incompletely-formed root with the inferior-alveolar neurovascular bundle is shown. H-E stain X15

Fig. 4-9-2 Transverse section of the root showing the root canal. H-E stain X15

1.	Dentin	**6.**	Vein
2.	Apical foramen	**7.**	Periodontal ligament
3.	Bone of the mandibular canal	**8.**	Secondary dentin
		9.	Predentin
4.	Inferior alveolar nerve	**10.**	Dental pulp
5.	Artery	**11.**	Blood vessel

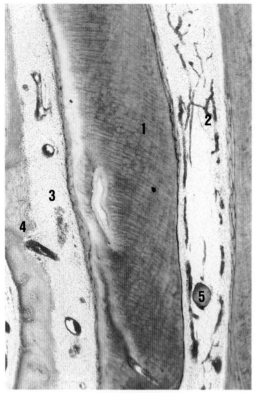

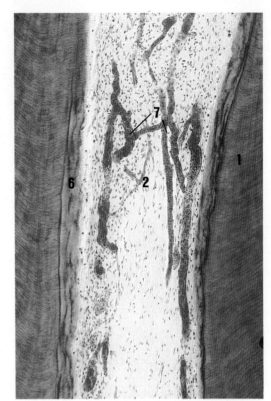

Fig. 4-10-1 Longitudinal section of the radicular pulp. A small denticle is evident within the root canal. H-E stain X40

Fig. 4-10-2 Longitudinal section of the radicular pulp. The anastomosis of blood vessels should be noted. H-E stain X80

1. Dentin
2. Radicular pulp
3. Periodontal ligament
4. Alveolar bone
5. Denticle
6. Secondary dentin
7. Blood vessel

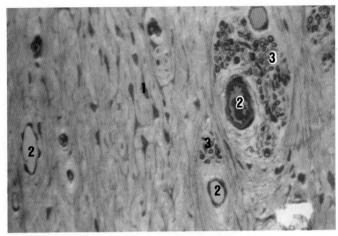

Fig. 4-11-1 Thin section of the dental pulp showing a small myelinated nerve. Toluidine blue stain X200

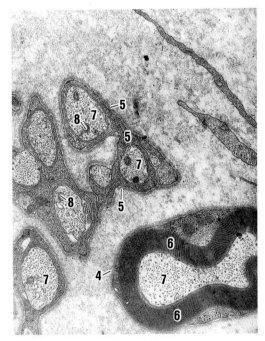

Fig. 4-11-2 Electron micrograph of myelinated and unmyelinated nerves in the pulp. X14,000

1.	Pulp cell	5.	Unmyelinated nerve fibers
2.	Blood vessel	6.	Myelin sheath
3.	Fascicle of nerve fibers	7.	Axon
4.	Myelinated nerve fiber	8.	Mitochondria

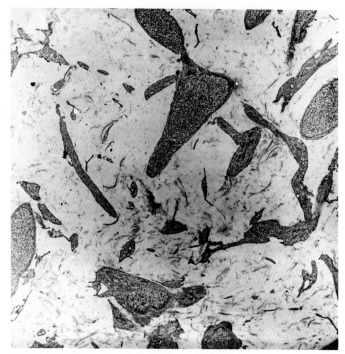

Fig. 4-12-1 Electron micrograph of fibroblasts in the pulp core. X4,500

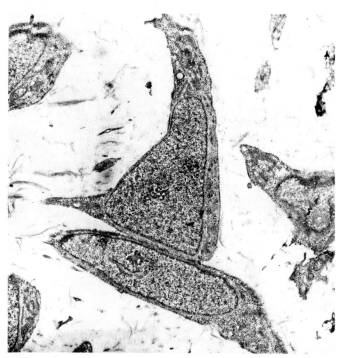

Fig. 4-12-2 Electron micrograph of fibroblasts in the pulp core. X8,000

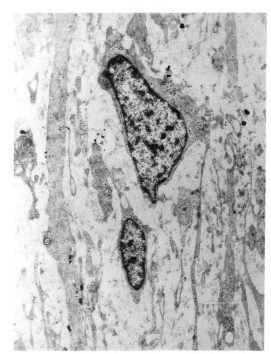

Fig. 4-13-1 Electron micrograph of cells in the pulp core. X4,500

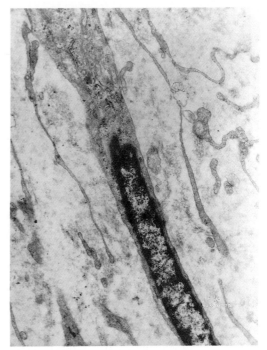

Fig. 4-13-2 Electron micrograph of a pulp cell. X8,000

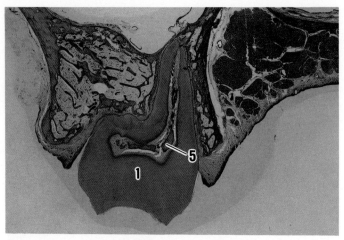

Fig. 4-14-1 Longitudinal section of a tooth showing the coronal and radicular pulp with denticles. H-E stain X3

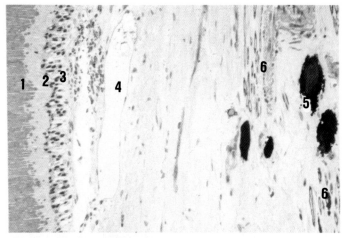

Fig. 4-14-2 Thin section of the radicular pulp showing small denticles. Toluidine blue stain X180

1. Dentin	**4.** Blood vessel
2. Predentin	**5.** Denticle
3. Odontoblastic layer	**6.** Nerve fibers

5

Tooth Structure: Cementum

TOOTH STRUCTURE: CEMENTUM

Cementum is a mineralized tissue that covers the entire root surface (Fig. 5-1-1). It is produced by cells of the dental follicle or sac called cementoblasts (Fig. 1-16-1, Fig. 1-19-2). It is similar to bone in several aspects: growth pattern, inorganic component, organic fibers, ground substance, and cellular arrangements.

Hertwig's epithelial root sheath is responsible for size, shape and number of roots formed. The stresses of eruption and the activity of root dentin formation may be contributing factors for the disruption of the root sheath. Consequently, the root sheath separates from the mineralized dentin surface and fragments. The remnants form the epithelial rests of Malassez (Fig. 1-31-2, Fig. 1-32-2). The ectomesenchymal cells of the dental follicle pass through the remnants of the root sheath and align against the calcified dentin. These cells become cementoblasts and produce the unmineralized matrix of cementum or cementoid. Cementum matrix is deposited in layers similar to bone. Periods of cementum formation are separated by resting or incremental lines. Some cementoblasts become incorporated into cementum as cementocytes. These cells reside within lacuna and maintain contact with the surface cells via cytoplasmic processes within canaliculi. Cementum differs from bone primarily by being avascular, continuously covered by a thin layer of cementoid, and deposited in lamellae at an extremely slow rate. These differences make the root more resistant to resorption than bone.

If a portion of the root sheath remains on the surface of the dentin, cementum will fail to form. Another possible consequence is the formation of an enamel pearl. This is a small nodule of hypomineralized, hypoplastic enamel on the root surface that most frequently occurs in the furcation of molar teeth.

About 60% of cementum is comprised of inorganic material in the form of hydroxyapatite crystals. The organic component is collagen and amounts to about 30% of cementum. About 10% of cementum is water. These percentages will vary depending on the age of the tooth and location of the sample on the root.

The fibrous component of cementum is unusual. The matrix contains small collagenous fibrils (intrinsic fibers) produced by the cementoblasts and large coarse bundles of collagen (extrinsic fibers) produced by the fibroblasts of the periodontal ligament. These large bundles are embedded extensions of the principal fiber bundles of the periodontal ligament (Fig. 5-5-2). The embedded portions are referred to as Sharpey's fibers. The principal fibers of the periodontal ligament are also embedded as Sharpey's fibers into alveolar bone. The two types of cementum based on the presence of cells are: acellular and cellular. Afibrillar cementum and intermediate cementum are also recognized.

Acellular or Primary Cementum

This type of cementum is formed without the inclusion of cells. It is the first-formed cementum and, as such, is part of the dentinocemental junction from the cementoenamel junction to the root apex. As a tissue, it is found predominately on the occlusal or cervical one-third of the root. However, it may be mixed with the cellular type in the middle one-third of the root. The incremental lines are very close together which indicates the extremely slow rate of formation. Numerous Sharpey's fibers are embedded into this cementum (Fig. 5-4-1). These extrinsic fibers are arranged more or less perpendicular to the cementum surface (Fig. 5-1-2, Figs. 5-5-1, 2). In demineralized, H-E stained sections, this type of cementum stains more basophilic or darker than the cellular type of cementum and can be easily distinguished from dentin (Fig. 5-8-1).

Cellular or Secondary Cementum

Cellular cementum contains buried cementocytes residing in lacunae (Figs. 5-3-1, 2). The long cytoplasmic processes of the cementocyte extend within canaliculi toward the periodontal ligament space (Figs. 5-2-1, 2). As a tissue, it is found primarily on the apical one-third of the root, especially around the apical foramen and within the furcation of molar teeth (Fig. 5-1-1). Thus the root surface may be lined by a mixture of acellular and cellular cementum (Fig. 5-5-1). Cellular cementum is formed more rapidly than acellular cementum. The incremental lines are more irregular and are spaced further apart (Fig. 5-6-2).

Afibrillar Cementum

In this type of cementum, the fibrillar component lacks the characteristic features of collagen. It is most commonly found along the cervical margin on the surface of the enamel. It may be formed by connective tissue cells of the dental follicle that gained access to the enamel surface following the local degeneration of the reduced enamel epithelium. This type has also been referred to as coronal cementum. If it persists, it is covered over by normal cementum (Fig. 5-6-1).

Intermediate Cementum

This type of cementum resembles dentin but without the presence of dentinal tubules. It is found between Tomes' granular layer in dentin and the dentinocemental junction (Fig. 3-19-1, Fig. 5-4-2). This tissue may not be present in all roots. Cellular elements may be found within this layer.

Cementoenamel Junction

The cementoenamel junction can exist in three different arrangements. In the most common junction (60%), the cementum overlies the enamel surface for a short distance (Fig. 5-6-1). Cementum may extend over enamel in the form of a cemental spur, especially in the furcation of molar teeth. In the second most common form (30%), the cementum and enamel meet in a relatively sharp line. In the least frequent junction (10%), the cementum and the enamel are separated by a short distance leaving a region of exposed dentin.

Dentinocemental Junction

This junction is easily distinguished by the deep basophilia in H-E stained sections. This is in contrast to ground sections. This junction is usually smooth and straight in secondary teeth (Figs. 5-8-1, 2).

Cementoclasia and Cemental Repair

Cementum responds to changes in function by apposition of new cementum matrix. However, in cases of excessive masticatory loading, pressure or disease, resorption of cementum can occur. Resorption of cementum is similar to that of bone. Active odontoclasts, similar to osteoclasts, resorb cementum where they reside in surface depressions (Howship's lacunae). At the end of the resorptive period, cementum formation will partially or completely repair the root surface. The cementum may be of either type or a combination of both. In some cases of extreme trauma, the cementum may be torn away from the surface of the dentin. Fragments are reattached by the formation of new cementum (Figs. 5-7-1, 2).

Cementosis and Cementicles

The formation of cementum occurs throughout the life of the tooth stimulated by masticatory function. However, hypercementosis may occur from the lack of function or inflammation (hyperplasia) or from an increase in physiologic function (hypertrophy).

Cementicles are small, irregular calcified bodies found in the periodontal ligament space near the root surface. They may be free within the periodontal ligament, attached to the root surface or embedded in the cementum (Figs. 5-8-1, 2).

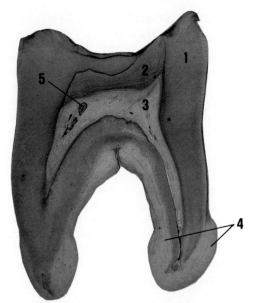

Longitudinal section of a demineralized molar. Hypertrophy of the cementum is seen at the root apex of both roots and within the furcation area. The reparative dentin in the roof of the pulp chamber should be noted.

Fig. 5-1-1 Demineralized longitudinal section of a human mandibular molar. H-E stain X5

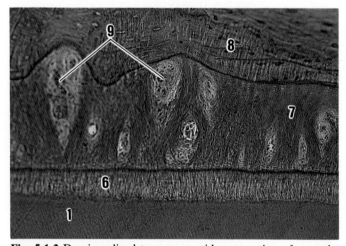

Sharpey's fiber can be seen within the acellular cementum and the alveolar bone.

Fig. 5-1-2 Demineralized transverse mid-root section of a tooth root. Azan stain X120

1. Dentin	6. Acellular cementum
2. Reparative dentin	7. Periodontal ligament
3. Dental pulp	8. Alveolar bone
4. Cementum	9. Interstitial space
5. Denticle	

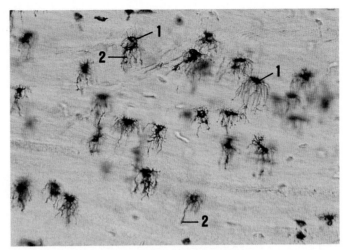

Fig. 5-2-1 Ground section showing cementocyte lacunae within cellular cementum. Silver impregnation (green filter) X90

Canaliculi radiate from the cementocyte lacuna. Most of the canaliculi extend toward the periodontal ligament space.

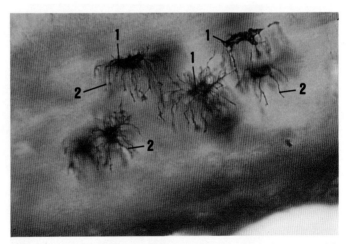

Fig. 5-2-2 Ground section showing cementocyte lacunae with canaliculi. Silver impregnation X720

1. Cementocyte lacuna   2. Cementocyte canaliculus

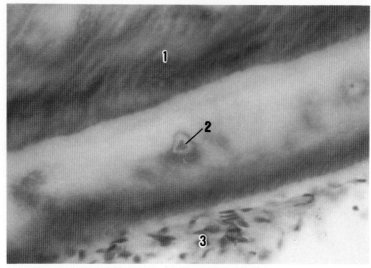

Fig. 5-3-1 Demineralized section of cellular cementum. H-E stain X400

1. Dentin   2. Cementocyte   3. Periodontal ligament

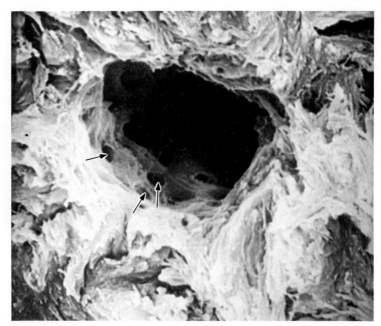

Fig. 5-3-2 Scanning electron micrograph of a cementocyte lacuna. Arrows indicate openings into canaliculus. X4,000

Transverse section of Sharpey's fibers (extrinsic fibers) among the network of fibrils (intrinsic fibers).

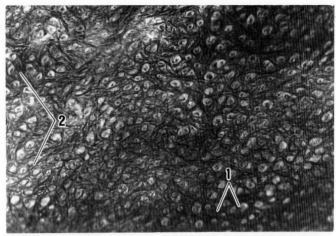

Fig. 5-4-1 Tangential section of acellular cementum showing a dense pattern of Sharpey's fibers. van Gieson stain X540

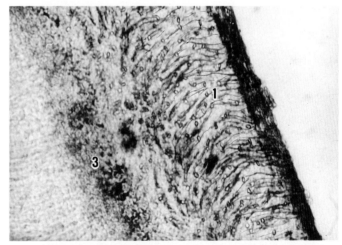

Fig. 5-4-2 Longitudinal ground section of cellular cementum. X180

1. Sharpey's fibers
2. Matrix of cementum fibrils
3. Tomes' granular layer

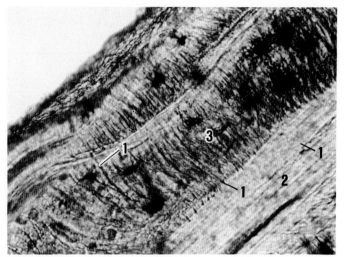

A layer of cellular cementum is seen on the surface of acellular cementum. The spacing between the incremental lines should be compared in both types of cementum.

Fig. 5-5-1 Ground section of root surface illustrating Sharpey's fibers. Silver impregnation-carbol fuchsin stain X180

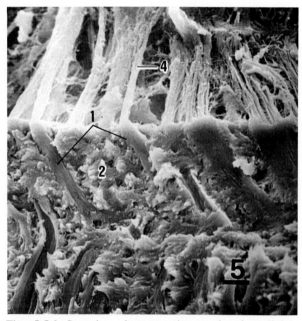

The portion of the principal fibers of the periodontal ligament embedded in cementum is referred to as a Sharpey's fiber.

Fig. 5-5-2 Scanning electron micrograph of acellular cementum and the principal fibers of the periodontal ligament. X6,000

1. Sharpey's fibers
2. Acellular cementum
3. Cellular cementum
4. Principal fibers of the periodontal ligament

The cervical area of the enamel is covered by cementum. This is the most common form of the cementoenamel junction.

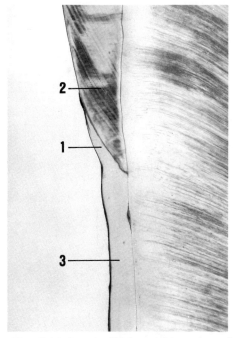

Fig. 5-6-1 Longitudinal ground section of a tooth at the cementoenamel junction. X80

Lamella in cellular cementum are of different widths. The irregular incremental lines are dark staining.

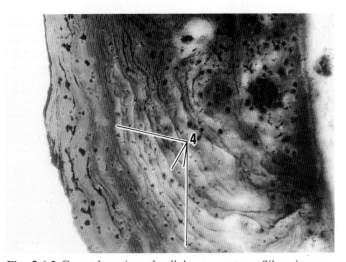

Fig. 5-6-2 Ground section of cellular cementum. Silver impregnation X80

1. Cementum spur	**3.** Acellular cementum
2. Enamel	**4.** Cellular cementum

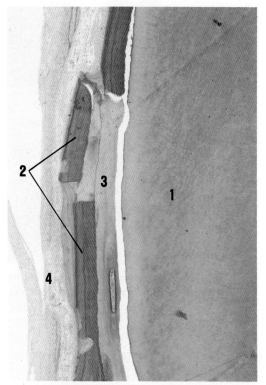

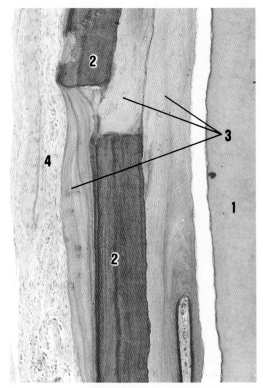

Fig. **5-7-1** Demineralized section showing the repair of torn cementum due to occlusal trauma in a mandibular canine of an 81-year-old person. H-E stain X80

Fig. **5-7-2** Enlargement of part of Fig. 5-7-1. X200

1. Dentin
2. Torn cementum
3. Region of cementum repair
4. Periodontal ligament

The dentinocemental junction is easily distinguished. Both types of cementum are present on the root surface. Embedded cementicles can be seen.

Cementicles can be attached to the root surface or free within the periodontal ligament.

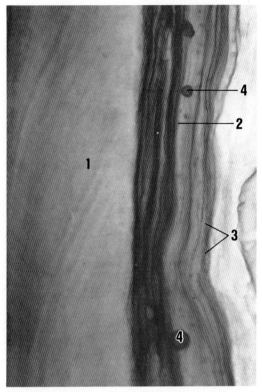

Fig. 5-8-1 Demineralized longitudinal section of tooth root. H-E stain X200

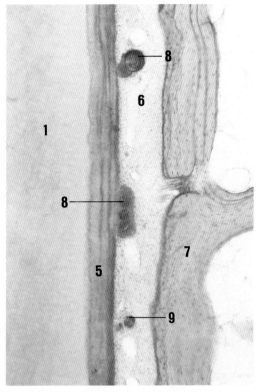

Fig. 5-8-2 Demineralized longitudinal section of tooth root. H-E stain X100

1. Dentin
2. Cellular cementum
3. Incremental lines
4. Embedded cementicle
5. Acellular cementum

6. Periodontal ligament
7. Alveolar bone
8. Attached cementicle
9. Free cementicle

6

Periodontium

PERIODONTIUM

The periodontium consists of the gingiva, periodontal ligament, alveolar bone and cementum. Functionally, it comprises those tissues that surround and support the tooth. The cementum, periodontal ligament and alveolar bone are called the supporting structures of the teeth.

Gingiva

The gingiva is that portion of the oral mucosa the surrounds the neck of the teeth and covers the margin of the alveolar bone (Fig. 6-1-1). The oral mucosa consists of stratified squamous epithelium (Figs. 6-19-1 to 6-21-2) supported by a fibrous lamina propria (Fig. 6-2-1, Fig. 6-16-1). The gingiva is attached to both the tooth and alveolar bone. The gingiva is separated from the alveolar mucosa by the mucogingival line except on the hard palate. The area of the gingiva above the crest of the alveolar bone is loosely attached and is referred to as the free or marginal gingiva (Fig. 6-2-1, Fig. 6-16-1). That portion of the gingiva that overlies the alveolar bone is more tightly bound and is referred to as the attached gingiva. These two regions are separated by the free gingival groove. The free gingiva is separated from the tooth surface by the gingival sulcus. The bottom of the gingival sulcus roughly corresponds to the level of the free gingival groove.

The oral surface of the free gingiva merges with the dento-gingival surface at the free gingival margin. The epithelium covering the free gingiva is designated as oral gingival epithelium, sulcular epithelium and junctional epithelium. The oral gingiva is keratinized or parakeratinized stratified squamous epithelium depending on functional abrasion. The sulcular epithelium is thinner and nonkeratinized. The junctional epithelium continues apically below the gingival sulcus and is attached directly to the enamel surface. Junctional epithelium originates from the reduced enamel epithelium of the enamel organ. The interface between the connective tissue and the regions of the marginal gingiva is variable. The oral surface shows numerous epithelial pegs and connective tissue papilla whereas the sulcular and junctional surfaces are relatively smooth (Fig. 6-16-1, Figs. 6-17-1, 2, 3).

The lamina propria of the gingiva is similar to dense fibrous connective tissue in other areas of the body. The fibroblast is the principal cell type. Mast cells and macrophages or histiocytes may also be found. Inflammatory cells, namely, neutrophilic granulocytes and lymphocytes are found in normal gingiva. These cells may pass through the sulcular epithelium to enter the gingival sulcus. The greatest bulk of the connective tissue fibers are collagen although elastic, reticular and oxytalin fibers may be found. The collagen fiber bundles within the gingiva are grouped together depending on their orientation or attachment. They are designated as circular, dentogingival, dentoperiosteal, and alveologingival fiber groups. The high content of collagen and a ground substance rich in glycosaminoglycans and glycoproteins, helps to maintain the firmness of the gingiva.

The blood vessels and nerves of the gingiva arises from three sources: periosteal, interdental and periodontal branches (Fig. 6-2-2, Figs. 6-18-1, 2, 3).

Periodontal Ligament

The periodontal ligament originates from the middle layer of the dental follicle. It is a specialized connective tissue that serves to attach the root surface to the alveolar bone (Fig. 6-1-2, Fig. 6-3-2, Fig. 6-5-2, Figs. 6-6-1, 2). It is continuous with the tissues of the gingiva, pulp, and marrow spaces (Fig. 6-3-1, Fig. 6-4-2, Fig. 6-12-2, Figs. 6-13-1, 2; Figs. 6-14-1, 2). The large bundles of connective tissue fibers are arranged together as principal fibers (Fig. 6-1-2, Fig. 6-3-2, Fig. 6-4-1, Fig. 6-7-2, Fig. 6-8-1, 2; Fig. 6-12-1). The principal fibers are classified according to their orientation or attachment: alveolar crest, horizontal, oblique, apical, interradicular. The transseptal fibers or the interdental ligament extends directly from tooth to tooth. The terminal ends of the principal fibers are deeply embedded into cementum and alveolar bone where they are called Sharpey's fibers (Fig. 5-5-2, Fig. 6-4-1, Fig. 6-7-2).

The principal cell in the periodontal ligament is the fibroblast. This cell is responsible for the synthesis and degradation of collagen (Fig. 6-8-2, Fig. 6-10-3). The cemental surface of the root is lined by cementoblasts for the production of cementum (Fig. 6-4-1). Within the periodontal ligament near the root, remnants of Hertwig's epithelial root sheath may be found. These are small cluster of epithelial cells known as epithelial rests of Malassez (Fig. 7-11-2, Fig. 6-15-1).

Blood and lymphatic vessels and nerves are found within areas of loose connective tissue referred to as interstitial spaces (Fig. 6-4-1, Fig. 6-8-1, Fig. 6-10-3). These spaces are found mainly near the bone surface between the principal fibers. Elastic fibers are confined to the walls of blood vessels. Reticular fibers aid in the support of the blood and lymphatic vessels and nerves. The oxytalin fiber extends from the superficial layer of cementum apically to terminate in association with blood vessels and nerves (Figs. 6-9-1, 2). The blood and nerve supply to the periodontal ligament arise from the dental artery and nerve. They enter the ligament space via perforating canals. There may be anastomosis with gingival blood vessels. Venous and lymph drainage follow a reverse course. The network of blood vessels together with the interstitial fluids assist the principal fibers in the resistance to apical displacement of the teeth under occlusal or masticatory loading. The two types nerves in the periodontal ligament are vasomotor for control of blood flow, and sensory for proprioception, pressure, and pain.

Alveolar Bone

The alveolar bone is that part of the maxilla and mandible that supports the roots of the teeth (Fig. 1-37-2, Figs. 6-1-1, 2). It consists of the alveolar bone proper and supporting bone. Each tooth resides within an alveolus or tooth socket, each of which are separated by interalveolar or interdental bone (Fig. 6-4-2, Figs. 6-5-1, 2; Fig. 6-7-1). The roots of multirooted teeth are separated by intra-alveolar or interradicular septa of bone (Fig. 6-1-2). The bone lining the alveoli is termed the alveolar bone proper. It is also referred to as the cribriform plate due to the numerous perforating nutrient channels (Volkman's canals), the lamina dura due to the radiographic appearance or the fibrous endosteum due to the fibers of the periodontal ligament, and bundle bone due to the large quantity of Sharpey's fibers (Fig. 6-7-2, Fig. 6-8-1, Fig. 6-10-1, 2; Fig. 6-15-1). It consists of lamellar bone which reflects the pattern of new bone apposition. The alveolar bone proper is supported by spongy bone with numerous marrow spaces and by cortical plates of compact bone (Figs. 6-13-1, 2). The cortical bone consists of Haversian systems or osteons and longitudinal lamellae. Osteons may be found in some areas of the alveolar bone proper (Fig 6-8-1). In the alveoli of the anterior teeth, the alveolar bone proper may be fused with the outer cortical plates (Fig. 6-1-1).

The alveolar crest is the most coronal border of the interdental septum. Laterally, it divides the alveolar bone proper from the cortical plates (Fig. 6-3-1, Fig. 6-7-1). Extending through the fundus or floor of the alveolus is a neurovascular canal which carries nerves and blood vessels to the pulp via the apical foramen (Fig. 6-13-2, Figs. 6-14-1, 2).

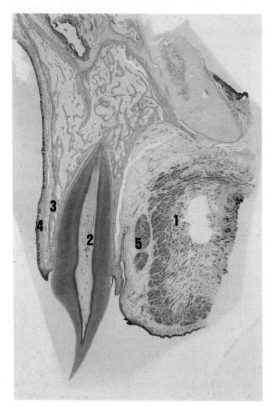

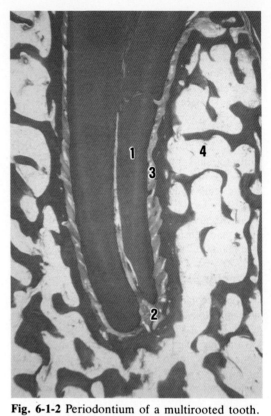

Fig. 6-1-1 Periodontium of the maxillary central incisor and the upper lip. H-E stain X5

1. Orbicularis oris muscle of upper lip 2. Maxillary central incisor 3. Alveolar bone, palatal side 4. Gingiva 5. Labial glands

Fig. 6-1-2 Periodontium of a multirooted tooth. H-E stain X8

1. Root of the tooth 2. Apical foramen 3. Periodontal ligament 4. Alveolar bone (interradicular septum)

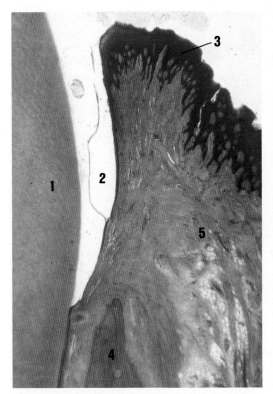

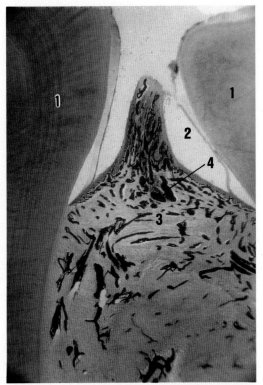

Fig. 6-2-1 Periodontium near the cervical margin of the tooth. H-E stain X25

1. Dentin 2. Gingival sulcus 3. Gingival epithelium 4. Alveolar bone (alveolar crest) 5. Lamina propria of the free gingiva

Fig. 6-2-2 Longitudinal section of the periodontium in the region of the interdental papilla near the cervical margin. van Gieson stain X6

1. Dentin 2. Enamel space 3. Lamina propria of interdental papilla 4. Blood vessel injected with India ink

Demineralization of the tooth removes the enamel. A fragment of the enamel cuticle from the surface of the enamel is present. The depth of the gingival sulcus and the length of the junctional epithelium can be seen.

The vascular supply of the interdental papilla shows the extensive distribution of blood vessels. The capillary plexus near the junctional epithelium should be noted.

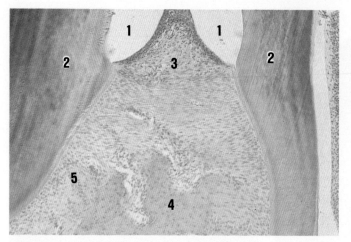

The alveolar crest is located about 1mm below the cementoenamel junction of the teeth. If the junctional epithelium moves apically onto the root surface, the height of the alveolar crest will be reduced accordingly. Neighboring teeth are connected by the transseptal fiber group.

Fig. 6-3-1 Longitudinal section of the cervical margin of neighboring teeth. PAS-Alcian blue stain X540

1. Enamel space 2. Dentin 3. Lamina propria of the interdental papilla 4. Crest of the alveolar bone 5. Periodontal ligament

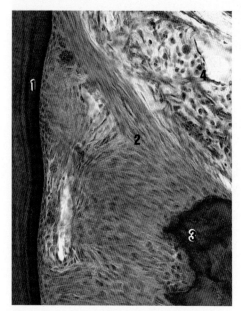

Two principal dentoalveolar fiber groups can be seen, the alveolar crest group and the cervical horizontal group.

Fig. 6-3-2 Longitudinal section of the cervical region of the periodontal ligament. H-E stain X360

1. Acellular (primary) cementum 2. Alveolar crest principal fiber group 3. Crest of the alveolar bone 4. Lamina propria of the free gingiva

The terminal ends of the horizontal fibers pass between the cementoblast and are embedded into cementum as Sharpey's fibers.

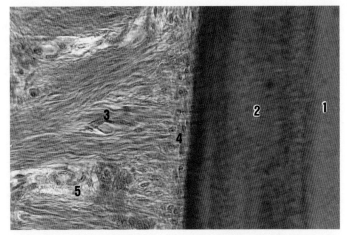

Fig. 6-4-1 Transverse section of the periodontal ligament. H-E stain X540

1. Dentin 2. Acellular (primary) cementum 3. Periodontal ligament 4. Cementoblast 5. Interstitial space

The interalveolar or interdental septum is perforated by passages that carry blood vessels and nerves. The marrow spaces are filled with adipose cells.

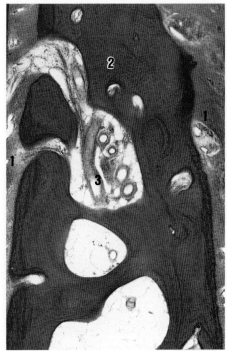

Fig. 6-4-2 Longitudinal section of alveolar bone. H-E stain X45

1. Periodontal ligament 2. Interalveolar or interdental septum 3. Blood vessel

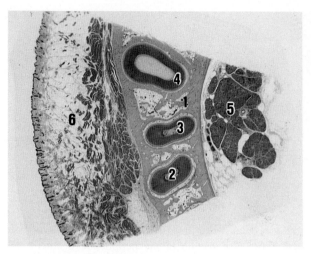

The transverse section of the mandible shows the roots of the incisors and the canine. The interalveolar septum and the cortical plates should be noted.

Fig. 6-5-1 Transverse section of the alveolar bone of the mandible. H-E stain X2
1. Alveolar bone with interdental septa and cortical plate 2. Root of mandibular central incisor 3. Root of mandibular lateral incisor 4. Root of mandibular canine 5. Sublingual gland 6. Cheek with buccinator muscle

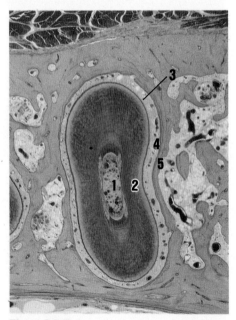

The cortical plates, alveolar bone proper, bone of the interdental septum, marrow spaces and alveolar blood vessels can be seen.

Fig. 6-5-2 Enlargement of mandibular lateral incisor in Fig. 6-5-1. H-E stain X4.5

1. Radicular pulp 2. Radicular dentin 3. Cementum 4. Periodontal ligament with interstitial spaces 5. Alveolar bone proper and marrow spaces

Epithelial rests of Malassez are visible in the periodontal ligament close to the cemental surface.

The distinct orientation of the principal fiber bundles can be seen between the interstitial spaces.

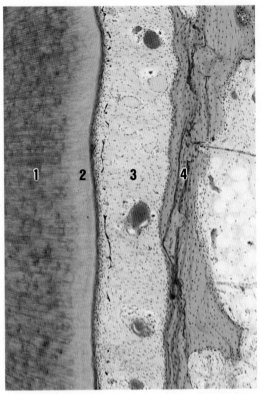

Fig. 6-6-1 Transverse section of the midroot region of a tooth. H-E stain X80

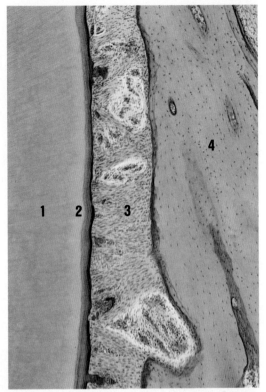

Fig. 6-6-2 Transverse section of the midroot region of a tooth. H-E stain X80

1. Dentin
2. Cementum

3. Periodontal ligament
4. Alveolar bone

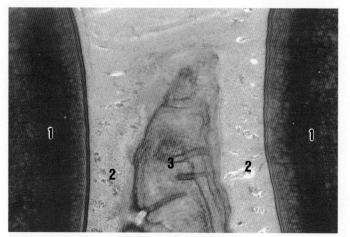

Fig. 6-7-1 Longitudinal section of crest of the alveolar bone. H-E stain X50

1. Dentin 2. Periodontal ligament 3. Crest of the alveolar bone

The crest of the alveolar bone is crossed by the transseptal fibers extending between two adjacent teeth.

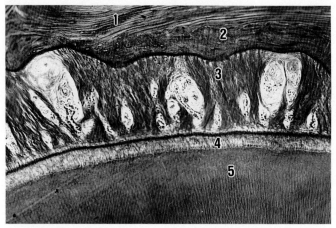

Fig. 6-7-2 Transverse section of the periodontal ligament. Silver impregnation X120

1. Lamellar bone 2. Bundle bone 3. Principal fiber group between interstitial spaces 4. Cementum 5. Dentin

The terminal ends of the principal fibers of the periodontal ligament are embedded into bone and cementum.

Principal fibers of the periodontal ligament are embedded into the alveolar bone proper. Sharpey's fibers do not occur within osteons.

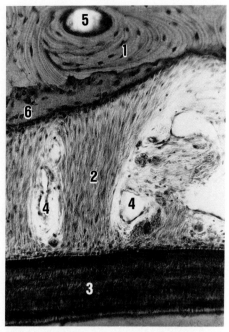

Fig. 6-8-1 Transverse section of the periodontal ligament. H-E stain X270

1. Lamellar bone of an osteon or Haversian system 2. Principal fibers of the periodontal ligament 3. Acellular cementum 4. Interstitial space 5. Haversian canal 6. Bundle bone

In a transverse section of a principal fiber bundle of the periodontal ligament, fibrocytes can be distinguished.

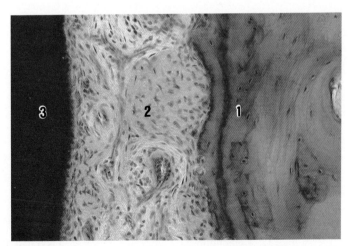

Fig. 6-8-2 Transverse section of the periodontal ligament. H-E stain X225

1. Alveolar bone 2. Principal fiber of the periodontal ligament 3. Cementum

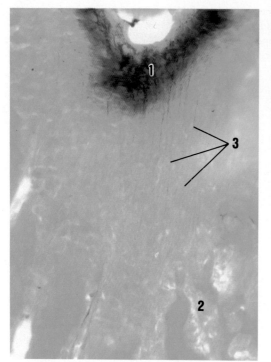

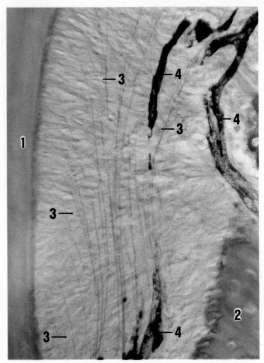

Fig. 6-9-1 Periodontal ligament of a mouse mandibular molar. Aldehyde fuchsin stain X300

Fig. 6-9-2 Periodontal ligament of a rat mandibular molar. Resorcin-fuchsin stain X600

Numerous oxytalan fibers, cut tangentially, arise from the cementum and pass into the periodontal ligament near the root apex.

Numerous oxytalan fibers extend apically from the surface layer of cementum toward blood vessels in the periodontal ligament.

1. Cementum
2. Alveolar bone
3. Oxytalan fibers
4. Blood vessel injected with India ink

146

Alveolar bone proper consists of lamellar bone and may contain a Haversian system. The numerous resting lines in the lamellar bone should be noted.

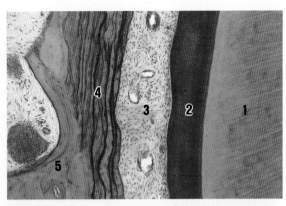

Fig. 6-10-1 Transverse section of the midroot region of a tooth. H-E stain X75

Blood vessels are located within the interstitial spaces. Osteoblasts and cementoblasts line the surface of the bone and the cementum respectively.

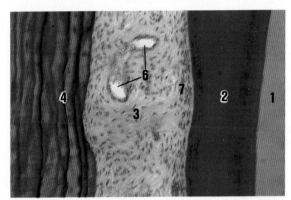

Fig. 6-10-2 Enlargement of part of Fig. 6-10-1. H-E stain X140

A blood vessel and a nerve fiber lie within the loose connective tissue of an interstitial space.

1. Dentin
2. Cementum
3. Periodontal ligament
4. Bundle bone
5. Lamellar bone
6. Blood vessel
7. Cementoblast
8. Nerve fiber bundle
9. Alveolar bone
10. Osteoblast

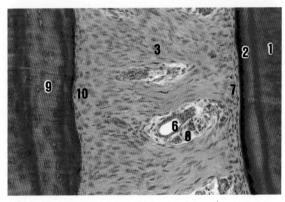

Fig. 6-10-3 Transverse section of the midroot region of a tooth. H-E stain X180

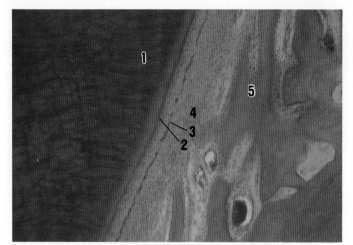

A strand of epithelial rests of Malassez is seen close to the cementum.

Fig. 6-11-1 Periodontal ligament of a tooth. H-E stain X90

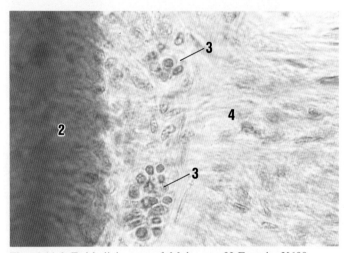

Small groups of epithelial cells comprise the rests of Malassez. They are found close to the root surface and are remnants of Hertwig's epithelial root sheath.

Fig. 6-11-2 Epithelial rests of Malassez. H-E stain X600

1. Dentin
2. Cementum
3. Epithelial rests of Malassez
4. Periodontal ligament
5. Alveolar bone

Bundles of collagen fibers extend from the cementum surface to form a plexus of fibers within the periodontal ligament.

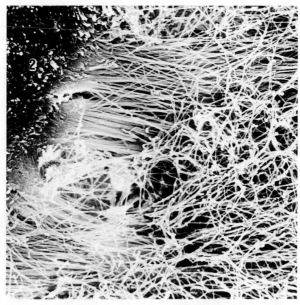

Fig. 6-12-1 Scanning electron micrograph of the cementum surface showing the principal fibers of the periodontal ligament. X3,600

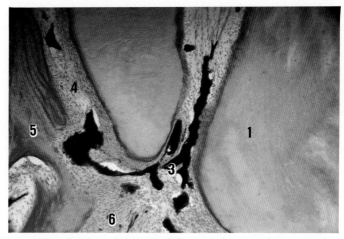

Fig. 6-12-2 Region of the apical foramen in a specimen vascular instilled with India ink. H-E stain X60

1.	Dentin	4.	Periodontal ligament
2.	Cementum	5.	Alveolar bone
3.	Blood vessel	6.	Neurovascular canal

The alveolar bone can be divided into the alveolar bone proper and supporting bone.

Nerve fibers and blood vessels which are distributed to the apical periodontal ligament and the pulp pass from the mandibular canal through the neurovascular canal.

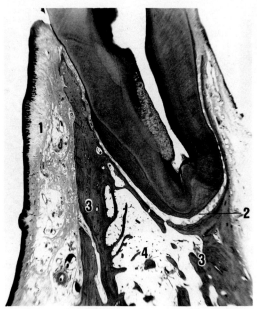

Fig. 6-13-1 Section of the alveolar bone. H-E stain X4

1. Attached gingiva 2. Periodontal ligament 3. Cortical plate of alveolar bone 4. Bone marrow space

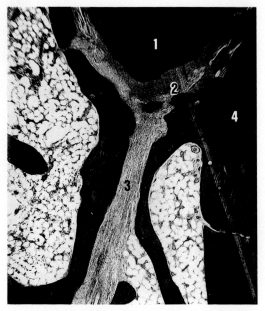

Fig. 6-13-2 Apical region of a tooth. H-E stain X8

1. Apex of the root 2. Periodontal ligament 3. Neurovascular canal 4. Alveolar bone

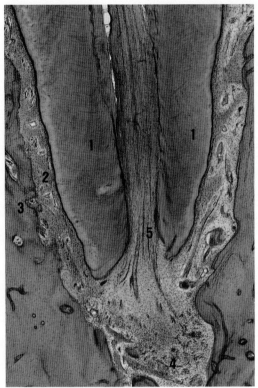

Fig. 6-14-1 Apical region of the root of a tooth. H-E stain X25

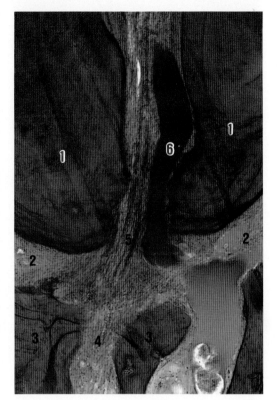

Fig. 6-14-2 Apical region of the root of a tooth. H-E stain X50

Nerve fibers can be seen entering the pulp through the apical foramen. Nerves and blood vessels supplying the pulp and the periodontal ligament are carried from the mandibular canal via the neurovascular canal through the floor of the alveolus.

The apical foramen is constricted by the deposition of cellular cementum.

1. Cementum
2. Periodontal ligament
3. Alveolar bone
4. Neurovascular canal
5. Nerve fiber bundle
6. Blood vessel

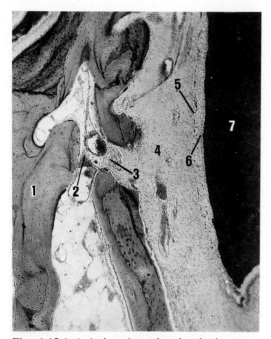

Fig. 6-15-1 Apical region of a developing root of a tooth. H-E stain X54

1. Alveolar bone 2. Blood vessel 3. Nerve fiber 4. Periodontal ligament 5. Epithelial rest of Malassez 6. Cementum 7. Dentin

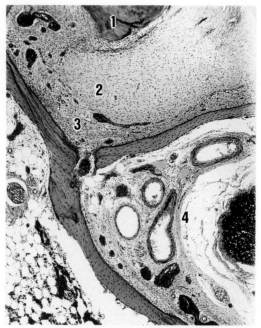

Fig. 6-15-2 Apical region of a developing root of a tooth. H-E stain X54

1. Apical region 2. Pulpal tissue in apical foramen 3. Periodontal ligament 4. Mandibular canal with inferior alveolar nerve and blood vessels

The pulpal tissue blends with the tissue of the periodontal ligament.

The numerous, long slender connective tissue papilla interdigitate with epithelial ridges to resist shear forces on the free and attached gingiva.

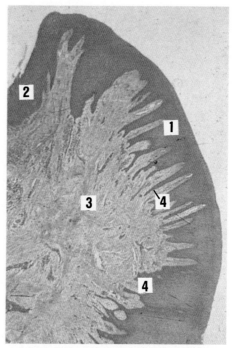

Fig. 6-16-1 Gingiva. H-E stain X70

1. Gingival epithelium 2. Gingival sulculus epithelium 3. Gingival lamina propria 4. Connective tissue papilla

The junctional epithelium is thinner with a smooth interface with the gingival lamina propria. The enamel space is bordered by the junctional epithelium and the dentin.

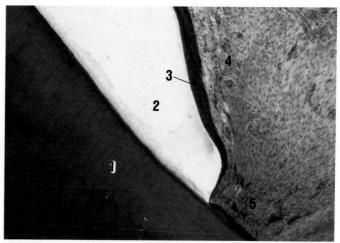

Fig. 6-16-2 Demineralized longitudinal section of the cervical margin of a tooth. H-E stain X90

1. Dentin 2. Enamel space 3. Junctional epithelium 4. Lamina propria 5. Cementum

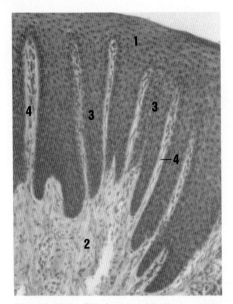

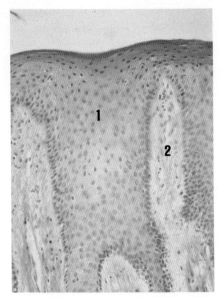

Fig. 6-17-1 Gingival epithelium. H-E stain X108

1. Gingival epithelium 2. Lamina propria 3. Epithelial ridge 4. Connective tissue papillae

The gingival epithelium is parakeratinized with numerous epithelial ridges interlocking with long slender connective tissue papilla.

Fig. 6-17-2 Gingival epithelium. H-E stain X225

1. Parakeratinized gingival epithelium 2. Connective tissue papilla

The characteristics of parakeratinized epithelium are the presence of pyknotic nuclei and keratin.

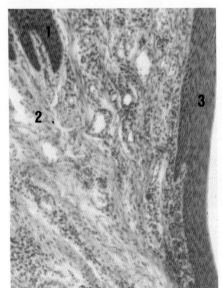

Fig. 6-17-3 Sulcular epithelium. H-E stain X108

1. Marginal epithelium 2. Lamina propria 3. Gingival sulcular epithelium

The epithelia of the gingival sulcus and the junctional epithelium are nonkeratinized.

The distribution of blood vessels within the lamina propria can be seen.

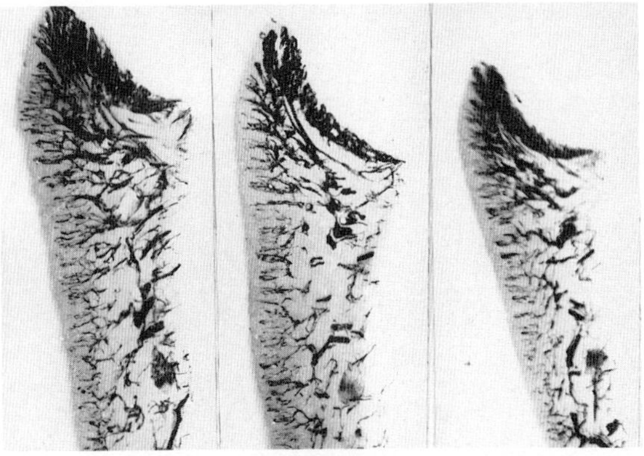

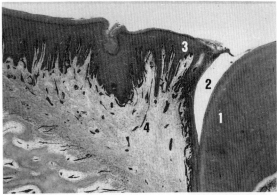

Fig. 6-18-1 Vascularly instilled human gingiva with India ink. H-E stain X10

Vascular distribution of the connective tissue papilla, lamina propria and bone are seen.

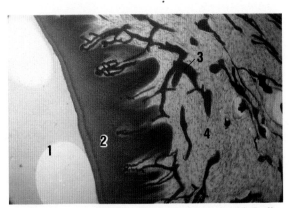

Fig. 6-18-2 Vascularly instilled dog gingiva with India ink. H-E stain X12

Capillary loops can be easily seen in the connective tissue papilla.

Fig. 6-18-3 Vascularly instilled dog gingiva with India ink. H-E stain X70

1. Gingival sulcus
2. Sulcular epithelium
3. Blood vessel
4. Lamina propria

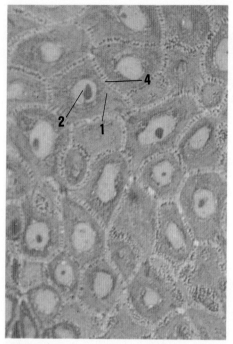

Fig. 6-19-1 Thin section of gingival epithelium. Toluidine blue stain X1,400

Intercellular bridges are seen between the cells of the stratum spinosum

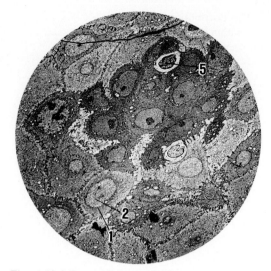

Fig. 6-19-2 Transmission electron micrograph of gingival epithelium. X1,000
Intercellular bridges are distinctive. Transient leukocyte is seen.

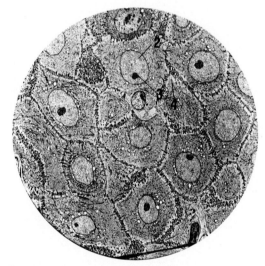

Fig. 6-19-3 Enlargement of Fig. 6-19-2. X1,500
Intercellular bridges are easily visible.

1. Gingival epithelial cell
2. Nucleus
3. Nucleolus
4. Intercellular bridges
5. Leukocyte

A migrating lymphocyte is seen between gingival epithelial cells.

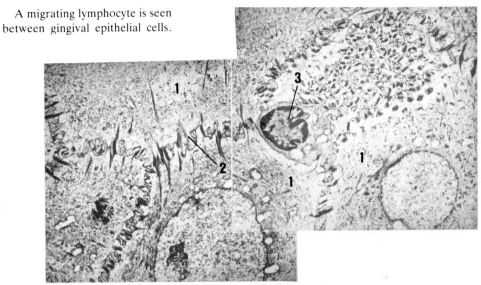

Fig. 6-20-1 Transmission electron micrograph composite of gingival epithelium with a transient lymphocyte. X2,700

Intercellular bridges are seen in transverse section.

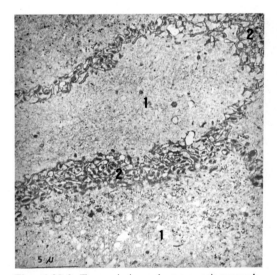

Fig. 6-20-2 Transmission electron micrograph of gingival epithelium. X4,500

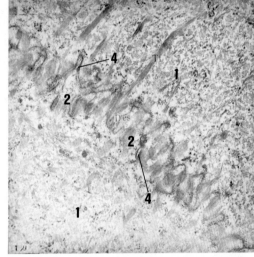

Fig. 6-20-3 Transmission electron micrograph of gingival epithelium. X10,000

Intercellular bridges are seen as interdigitating cell projections united by desmosomes (macula adherens).

1. Gingival epithelial cell
2. Intercellular bridges
3. Lymphocyte
4. Desmosomes

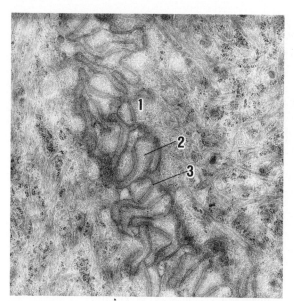

Fig. 6-21-1 Transmission electron micrograph of intercellular bridges. X18,000

The interdigitating cellular projections are called intercellular bridges.

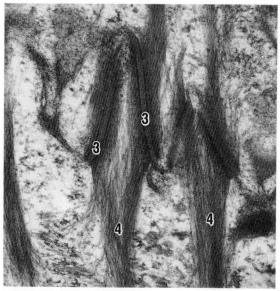

Fig. 6-21-2 Transmission electron micrograph of intercellular bridges. X45,000

Tonofilaments attach to an inner membrane plaque of the desmosome.

1. Gingival epithelial cell
2. Intercellular bridges
3. Desmosomes
4. Tonofibrils

7
Salivary Glands

SALIVARY GLANDS

The salivary glands are derived from the primitive oral ectoderm under the direction of the ectomesenchyme. The glands can be classified by different criteria, that is, by size, composition of the secretory units, and their duct system. By size, there are three major salivary glands, designated as the parotid, submandibular, and sublingual. There are numerous minor glands, including the labial, buccal, palatine, anterior lingual, glands of von Ebner and posterior lingual glands in the base of the tongue (Figs. 7-1-1 to 7-3-2). By the type of cells that comprise their secretory units, there are pure serous, pure mucous and mixed glands. According to the pattern of the duct system, salivary glands are classified as compound alveolar (acinar) or compound tubuloalveolar exocrine glands. The method of release of the secretory produce by both serous and mucous cells may vary between glands, and may depend on the nature and intensity of the secretory stimulus. The merocrine method of release is generally characteristic of these glands.

The salivary glands can be divided structurally into the parenchyma or secretory portion and the stroma or supportive portion. The latter is comprised of an enclosing capsule and supportive connective tissue partitions or septa that divide the gland into lobes and/or lobules.

The epithelium of the duct system begins as squamous to cuboidal cells, changes to pseudostratified columnar, then finally to stratified squamous epithelium near the oral mucosa.

Major Salivary Glands

Parotid

The parotid gland is the largest of the salivary glands. It is located anterior to the ear and overlies the masseter muscle (Fig. 7-1-1). It is designated as a pure serous gland, though it may contain some mucous cells in the newborn. The secretory units are in the form of tightly packed serous cells grouped together into alveoli or acini. These cells are pyramidal in shape with round basal nuclei, well-developed rough endoplasmic reticulum and Golgi complexes (Fig. 7-6). The apical portions are filled with secretory or zymogen granules (Figs. 7-7-1, 2). The parotid produces the enzyme salivary amylase (ptyalin) and some glycoproteins. Based on their production of glycoproteins, the secretory cells have been classified as seromucous.

The serous cells and the cells of the first segment of the duct system are enclosed by special stellate-shaped, contractile cells referred to as myoepithelial cells. These cells are thought to be derived from epithelial stem cells. Their long processes, which contain smooth muscle-like myofilaments, course outside the basal lamina next to the secretory cells. Contraction of these cells is thought to facilitate the discharge of the secretory products from the alveoli.

The salivary secretions pass through a series of ducts in route to the oral cavity and include the intralobular (intercalated and striated), interlobular and lobar ducts. The first segment of the intralobular duct system are the long, thin intercalated ducts composed of secretory cuboidal cells (Fig. 7-8-2). The second segment is composed of cuboidal-to-columnar striated duct cells characterized by basal striations and numerous elongated mitochondria (Figs. 7-4-1, 2; Figs. 7-5-1, 2). These ducts are usually surrounded by capillaries and are thought to function in ionic transport. The interlobular ducts are located between the lobules and are surrounded by connective tissue. They are lined by columnar epithelium. The main excretory duct, Stenson's duct, exits the gland at the anterior corner of the gland and runs forward, turns around the anterior border of the masseter muscle, pierces the buccinator muscle and mucous membrane of the cheek to open into the oral cavity via the parotid papilla opposite the maxillary second molar (Fig. 7-1-1).

The parotid gland is surrounded by a thick connective tissue capsule and extensive, well-developed septa. The connective tissue septa divide the parotid gland into lobes and lobules. Branches of the facial nerve pass through the gland within the connective tissue stroma. Adipose cells are frequently seen within the connective tissue septa (Figs. 7-4-1, 2). The amount of fat within the connective tissue increases with advancing age.

Submandibular gland

The submandibular gland is the second largest salivary gland and is designated as a mixed seromucous gland (about one-fourth mucous cells and three-fourths serous cells). The gland is located in the submandibular triangle, posterior and inferior to the mylohyoid muscle. The secretory cells are found in two arrangements, as pure serous alveoli and as caps or demilunes of serous cells on the terminus of mucous alveoli (Fig. 7-9-3, Figs. 7-10-1, 2; Figs. 7-11-1, 2; Figs. 7-12-1, 2). Both arrangements include the presence of myoepithelial cells (Fig. 7-13-2). The serous cells have well-developed rough endoplasmic reticulum, Golgi complexes and secretory granules (Figs. 7-12-1, 2). The mucous cells feature an oval nuclei compressed against the base of the cell. The apical portion is filled with mucigen granules.

The intercalated duct segments are fewer in number and shorter than in the parotid gland, whereas the striated ducts are much longer. The striated duct cells feature numerous mitochondria in the basal part of the cell (Fig. 7-13-1). The main excretory duct, Wharton's duct, courses along the superior surface of the mylohyoid muscle toward the midline to enter the oral cavity via the sublingual papilla or caruncula sublingualis at the side of the lingual frenulum in the floor of the mouth (Fig. 7-1-2, Figs. 7-2-1, 2).

The stoma consists of a well-developed connective tissue capsule and prominent connective tissue partitions.

Sublingual glands

The sublingual gland is the smallest of the major salivary glands. It is classified as a mixed seromucous gland, roughly one-third serous cells and two-thirds mucous cells (Figs. 7-14-1, 2). The serous secretory cells are found only in the form of serous demilunes (Fig. 7-15-2, Figs. 7-16-1, 2). The composition of the mucous secretory vacuoles may vary (Figs. 7-17-1, 2). Some mucous cells (Type I) produce both neutral and acidic glycoproteins while others (Type II) produce only acidic glycoproteins (Fig. 7-16-3). The sublingual gland contains both cell types of mucous cells, whereas the submandibular gland contains predominately Type II mucous cells. The gland is located between the oral mucosa and the lateral attachment of the mylohyoid muscle and contributes to the formation of the sublingual fold.

The intralobular ducts are poorly developed or even absent. Hence, the alveoli empty directly into secretory tubules (Figs. 7-14-1 to 7-16-2). The main excretory duct, Bartholin's duct, joins the submandibular duct and empties into the oral cavity through the sublingual papilla. In addition, a series of 6-12 small ducts may open directly into the oral cavity along the sublingual fold (Fig. 7-2-1).

The sublingual gland is enclosed by a thin connective tissue capsule. The gland, however, is partitioned by distinctive connective tissue septa (Fig. 7-14-1, Fig. 7-15-1).

Minor Salivary Glands

The minor salivary glands are found in most areas of the oral cavity. They reside within the lamina propria or submucosa of the oral mucosa (Fig. 7-2-2, Figs. 7-3-1, 2). Their glycoprotein-rich products empty into the oral cavity by way of short ducts. The anterior lingual, labial and buccal are considered to be seromucous glands (Figs. 8-2-1, 2; Figs. 8-9-1, 2). The posterior lingual, palatine and glossopalatine are designated as pure mucous. Only the glands of von Ebner are considered to be pure serous in composition (Figs. 9-10-1, 2).

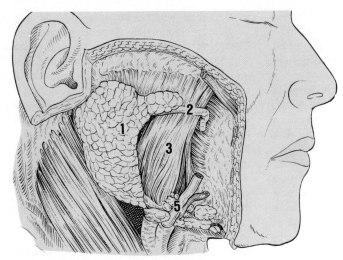

Fig. 7-1-1 Diagram of the parotid gland

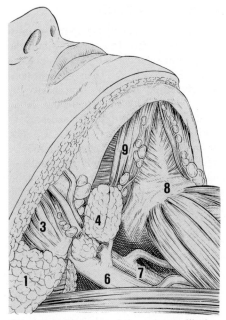

Fig. 7-1-2 Diagram of the submandibular gland

1. Parotid gland
2. Parotid gland duct (Stenson)
3. Masseter muscle
4. Submandibular gland
5. Facial vein
6. Internal jugular vein
7. External carotid artery
8. Hyoid bone
9. Digastric muscle (anterior belly)

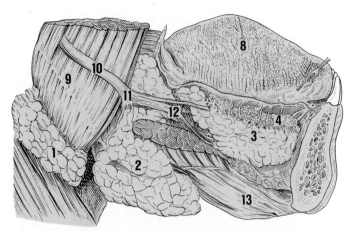

Fig. 7-2-1 Diagram of the submandibular and sublingual glands

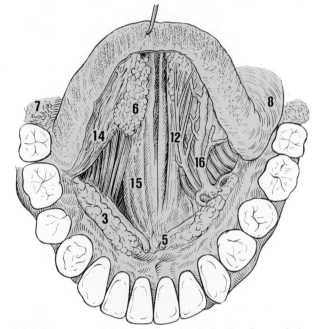

Fig. 7-2-2 Diagram of the salivary glands in the floor of the oral cavity

1. Parotid gland
2. Submandibular gland
3. Sublingual gland
4. Minor sublingual gland ducts
5. Submandibular gland duct (Wharton)
6. Anterior lingual gland
7. Retromolar glands
8. Tongue
9. Masseter muscle
10. Lingual nerve
11. Submandibular ganglion
12. Hypoglossal nerve
13. Digastric muscle (anterior belly)
14. Styloglossus muscle
15. Genioglossus muscle
16. Lingual vein

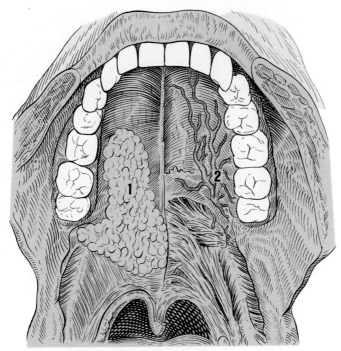

Fig. 7-3-1 Diagram of the palatine glands.

1. Palatine glands 2. Major palatine artery

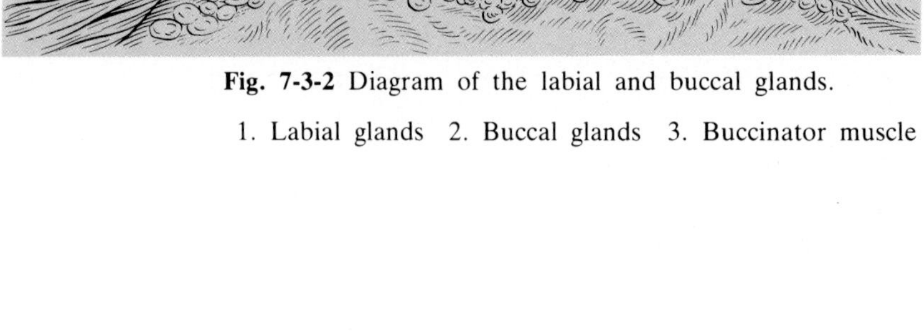

Fig. 7-3-2 Diagram of the labial and buccal glands.

1. Labial glands 2. Buccal glands 3. Buccinator muscle

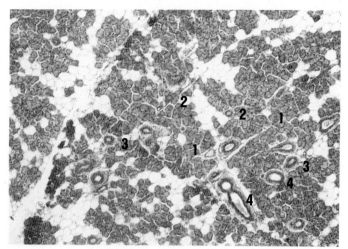

Fig. 7-4-1 Parotid gland. H-E stain X180

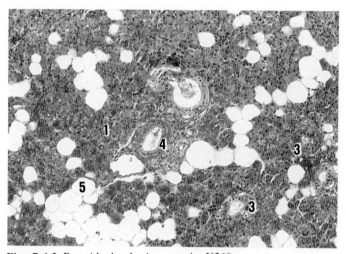

Fig. 7-4-2 Parotid gland. Azan stain X360

1. Serous or seromucous alveolus
2. Intercalated duct
3. Striated duct
4. Interlobular excretory duct
5. Adipose cell

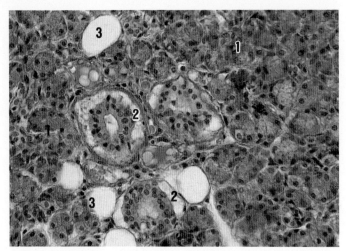

Fig. 7-5-1 Parotid gland. H-E stain X400

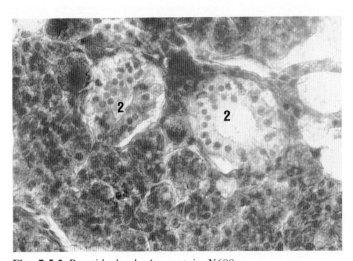

Fig. 7-5-2 Parotid gland. Azan stain X600

---

1. Serous or seromucous alveolus   **3.** Adipose cell
2. Striated duct

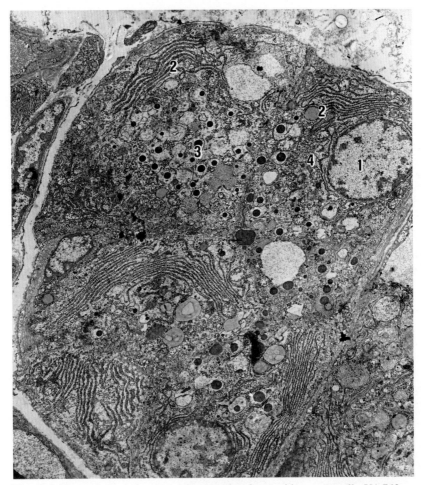

Fig. 7-6 Transmission electron micrograph of parotid serous cell. X1,760

1. Nucleus
2. Granular (rough) endoplasmic reticulum
3. Secretory granules
4. Golgi complexes

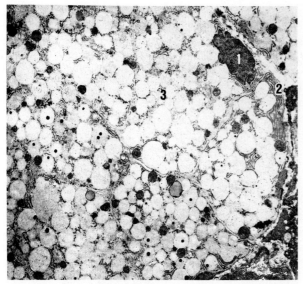

Fig. 7-7-1 Transmission electron micrograph of parotid gland (Macaca fuscata). X4,800

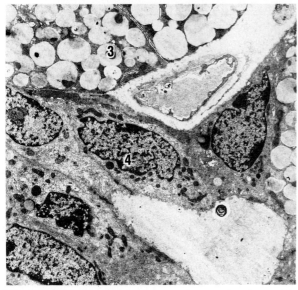

Fig. 7-7-2 Transmission electron micrograph of parotid gland (Macaca fuscata) X6000

1. Nucleus	3. Secretory (zymogen) granules in serous cell
2. Golgi complex	4. Nucleus of intercalated duct cell

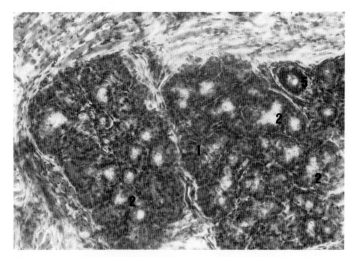

Fig. 7-8-1 Submandibular gland. H-E stain X450

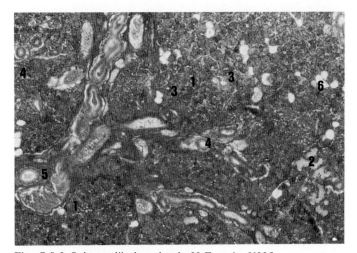

Fig. 7-8-2 Submandibular gland. H-E stain X225

1. Serous alveoli
2. Mucous cells with serous cells
3. Intercalated duct
4. Striated duct
5. Interlobular excretory ducts
6. Adipose cells

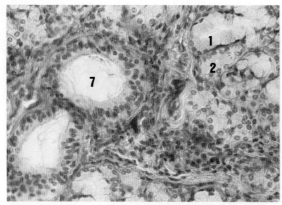

Fig. 7-9-1 Submandibular gland. Azan stain X330

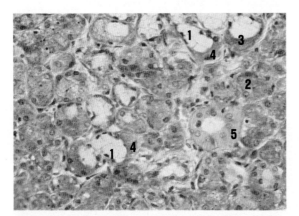

Fig. 7-9-2 Submandibular gland. Azan stain X330

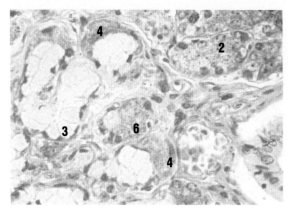

Fig. 7-9-3 Submandibular gland. Azan stain X330

1. Mucous cells
2. Serous cells
3. Mixed alveolus
4. Serous demilune
5. Striated duct
6. Secretory (zymogen) granules
7. Interlobular excretory duct

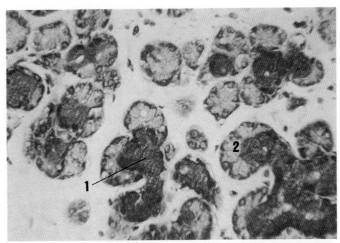

Fig. 7-10-1 Submandibular gland. Toluidine blue stain X400

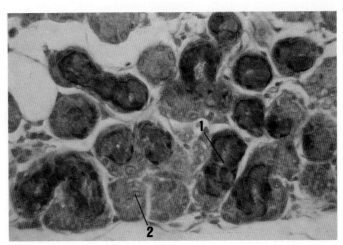

Fig. 7-10-2 Submandibular gland. Alcian green-metanil-yellow stain X400

1. Mucous cell
2. Serous cell

171

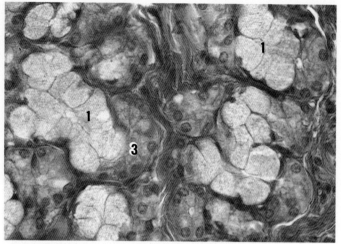

Fig. 7-11-1 Mixed alveolus of the submandibular gland. H-E
stain X900

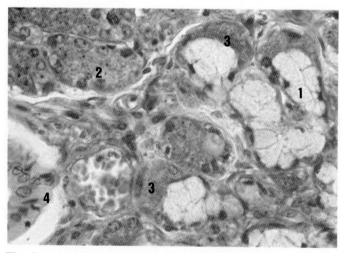

Fig. 7-11-2 Submandibular gland. Azan stain X1,170

1. Mucous cells
2. Mixed alveolus
3. Serous demilune
4. Striated duct

172

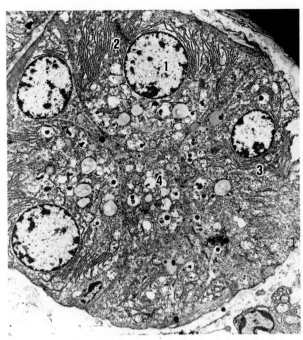

Fig. 7-12-1 Transmission electron micrograph of serous alveolus in the submandibular gland. X3,500

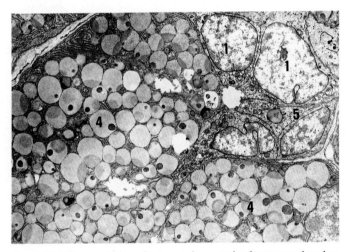

Fig. 7-12-2 Transmission electron micrograph of mucous alveolus in the submandibular gland (Macaca fuscata). X4,500

1. Nucleus
2. Granular (rough) endoplasmic reticulum
3. Golgi complex

4. Secretory (mucigen) granules in mucous cell
5. Intercalated duct cell

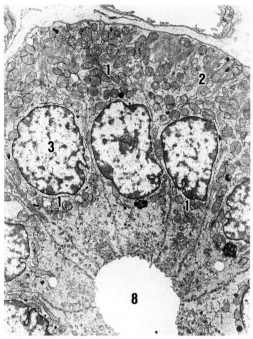

Fig. 7-13-1 Transmission electron micrograph of striated duct in the submandibular gland (Macaca fuscata). X3,500

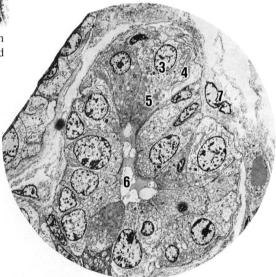

Fig. 7-13-2 Transmission electron micrograph of mixed alveolus in the developing submandibular gland (Human fetus). X2,250

1. Mitochondria	5. Secretory granules of mucous cell
2. Basal infolding	6. Lumen of secretory alveolus
3. Nucleus	7. Nucleus of myoepithelial cell
4. Golgi complex	8. Lumen of striated duct

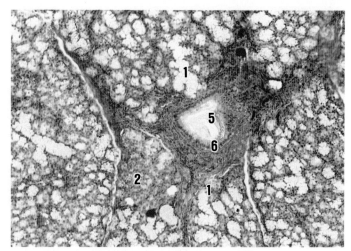

Fig. 7-14-1 Sublingual gland. Azan stain X360

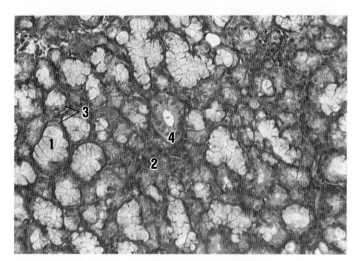

Fig. 7-14-2 Sublingual gland. H-E stain X360

1. Mucous alveolus	**4.** Striated duct
2. Serous alveolus	**5.** Interlobular excretory duct
3. Serous demilune	**6.** Interlobular connective tissue septa

175

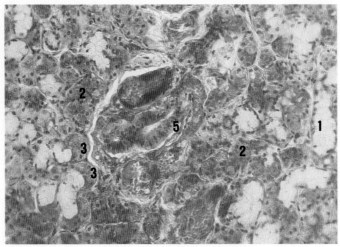

Fig. 7-15-1 Sublingual gland. Azan stain X360

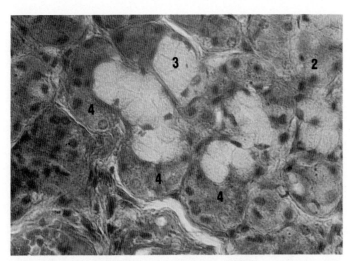

Fig. 7-15-2 Sublingual gland. Azan stain X540

1. Mucous alveolus
2. Serous alveolus
3. Mixed seromucous alveolus
4. Serous demilune
5. Interlobular excretory duct

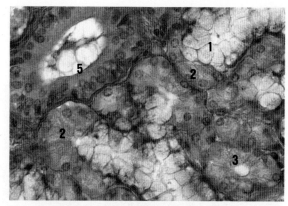

Fig. 7-16-1 Sublingual gland. H-E stain X750

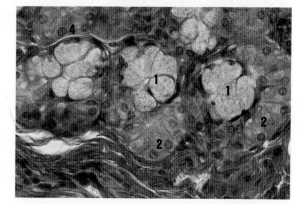

Fig. 7-16-2 Sublingual gland. H-E stain X900

Mucous cells within the sublingual gland produce both neutral and acidic glycoproteins. These two types of mucous cells can be distinguished by using an Alcian blue stain at a low pH.

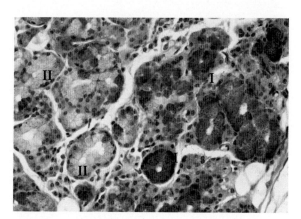

Fig. 7-16-3 Two types of mucous cells (I and II) can be seen in the sublingual gland (Macaca fuscata). The deeply stained cells are Type I cells. Alcian blue (pH 0.5) X750

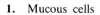

1. Mucous cells
    I. Type I mucous cells
    II. Type II mucous cells
2. Serous demilune
3. Intercalated duct
4. Interlobular duct

The secretory granules of the serous cells in the sublingual gland are coreless.

In Type I mucous cells of the sublingual gland, the granules appear fused.

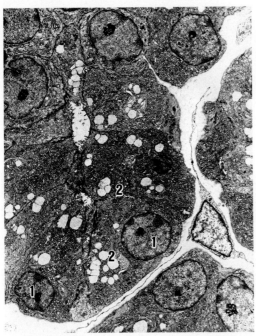

Fig. 7-17-1 Transmission electron micrograph of seromucous cell in the sublingual gland (Macaca fuscata). X1,800

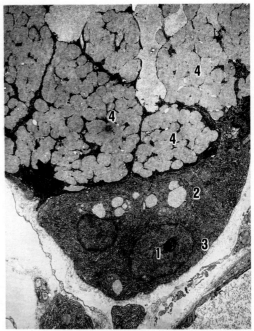

Fig. 7-17-2 Transmission electron micrograph of mucous cell and serous demilune cells in the sublingual gland (Macaca fuscata). X2,700

1. Nucleus
2. Secretory granules in seromucous cell
3. Serous demilune
4. Secretory (mucigen) granules in mucous cell (Type I)

8

Lips and Cheeks

LIPS AND CHEEKS

Lips

The lips of humans are characterized by the presence of a broad zone of transition between the mucosa of the oral cavity and the thin, hairy skin on the external surface. This zone is referred to as the red or vermillion border or the mucocutaneous junction. The outer surface is typical thin skin featuring a thin keratinized epidermis supported by a connective tissue dermis with hair follicles, sebaceous glands and sweat glands. The epidermis and dermis contain numerous sensory nerve endings which accounts for the acute sensitivity of the lips (Figs. 8-3-1, 2). The oral surface is covered by nonkeratinized stratified squamous epithelium with a lamina propria that blends with the dermis. In addition there is a submucosa containing the mixed seromucous labial glands (Figs. 8-2-1, 2). Between the oral mucosa and the skin is the orbicularis oris muscle that forms the core of the lips. This skeletal muscle functions to close, protrude and purse the lips and to press them against the teeth (Fig. 8-1-1 to Fig. 8-2-2).

The vermillion border is covered by a very thin keratinized epithelium that is semitransparent. The interface with the connective tissue features numerous, long vascular papillae extending close to the surface. The blood is carried near the surface and accounts for the reddish color of this zone.

Cheeks

The features of the cheek are similar to those of the lips. However, the buccinator muscle replaces the orbicularis oris muscle between the covering skin and the inner oral mucous membrane. The submucosa beneath the oral mucosa contains numerous mixed buccal seromucous salivary glands. Secretory alveoli may extend deep among the fascicles of the buccinator muscle. The glands empty into the buccal vestibule through short secretory ducts (Fig. 8-4-1 to Fig. 8-5-2). In addition to the minor salivary glands, ectopic sebaceous glands referred to as Fordyce spots or granules are also found within the oral mucosa of the cheeks. These yellowish-appearing glands are found in most adults and are not pathologic in nature.

In the retromolar triangle, there is a pad of tissue containing adipose connective tissue and minor seromucous salivary glands called retromolar glands. Within the check, near the parotid papilla, other minor salivary glands may be found. These molar glands are mixed seromucous although mucous cells predominate (Figs. 8-6-1, 2).

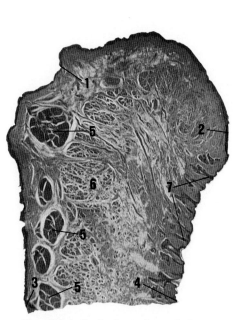

Fig. 8-1-1 Sagittal section of the lip. H-E stain X9.5

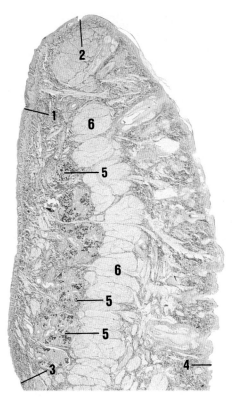

Fig. 8-1-2 Sagittal section of the lip (Macaca fuscata). PAS stain X5.5

1↔3. Oral mucous membrane
1↔2. Vermillion border
        (mucocutaneous junction)
2↔4. Thin skin

5. Labial seromucous glands
6. Orbicularis oris muscle
7. Hair follicles

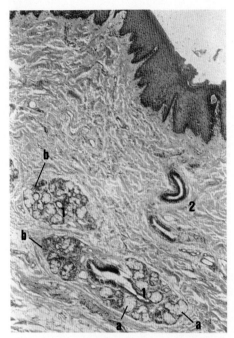

Fig. 8-2-1 Labial seromucous glands (Macaca fuscata). H-E stain X180

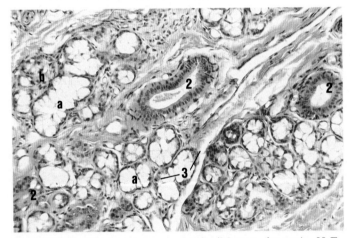

Fig. 8-2-2 Labial seromucous glands (Macaca fuscata). H-E stain X380

1. Labial seromucous glands
   a. Mucous alveolus
   b. Seromucous alveolus

2. Excretory duct
3. Serous demilune

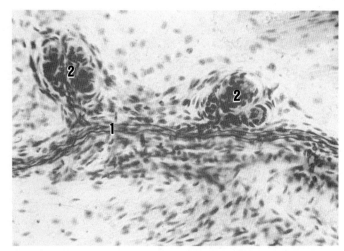

Fig. 8-3-1 Sensory nerve ending of the lip. Silver impregnation X800

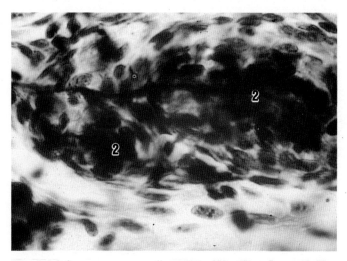

Fig. 8-3-2 Sensory nerve ending of the lip. Silver impregnation X1,200

---

1. Fascicle of nerve fibers   2. Nerve corpuscle of Golgi-Mazzoni

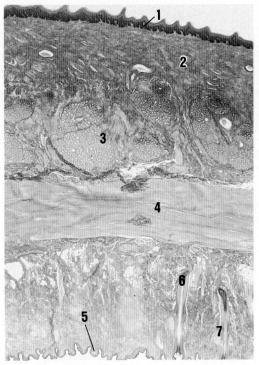

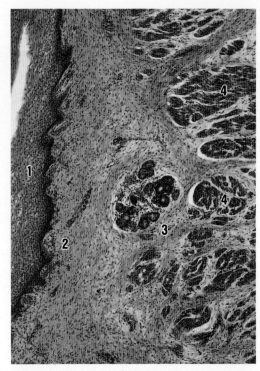

Fig. 8-4-1 Cheek (Macaca fuscata). H-E stain X40

Fig. 8-4-2 Frontal section of the buccal mucosa of a 17-week human fetus. H-E stain X1,000

1. Stratified squamous epithelium of buccal mucosa
2. Lamina propria of the oral mucosa
3. Buccal seromucous glands
4. Buccinator muscle
5. Epidermis
6. Hair
7. Sebaceous gland associated with a hair follicle

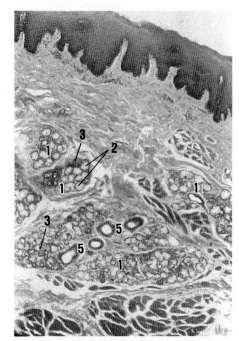

Fig. 8-5-1 Buccal glands (Macaca fuscata). H-E stain X70

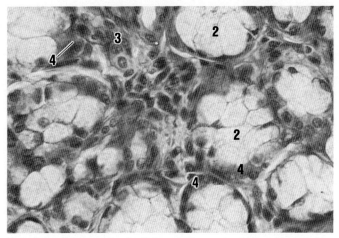

Fig. 8-5-2 Buccal glands (Macaca fuscata). H-E stain X1,000

1. Buccal seromucous glands
2. Mucous alveolus
3. Seromucous alveolus
4. Serous demilune
5. Excretory duct

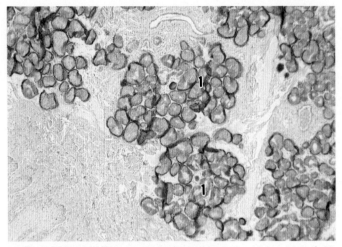

Fig. 8-6-1 Retromolar gland (Macaca fuscata). Alcian blue (pH 1.0) X160

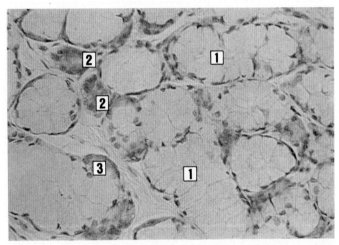

Fig. 8-6-2 Retromolar gland (Macaca fuscata). H-E stain X800

1. Mucous alveolus
2. Seromucous alveolus
3. Serous demilune

9
Tongue

TONGUE

The tongue is formed by a mixture of both extrinsic and intrinsic skeletal muscles (Fig. 9-1-2, Figs. 9-2-1, 2). The extrinsic muscles include the styloglossus, palatoglossus, genioglossus, hyoglossus and chondroglossus. The intrinsic muscles of the tongue are arranged in four groups: superior longitudinal fibers, transverse fibers, vertical fibers, and inferior longitudinal fibers (Fig. 9-3-1, 2). The motor innervation of the tongue is by the hypoglossal nerve or cranial nerve XII.

The dorsal surface of the anterior two-thirds or body of the tongue is covered by a specialized stratified squamous epithelium formed into small papillae, namely, filiform, fungiform, and circumvallate. Rudimentary foliate papillae are found on the lateral margins of the tongue. The lamina propria is bound tightly to the intrinsic muscles of the tongue. A submucosa is not present. The mucosa of the posterior one-third or root of the tongue is covered by numerous small elevations referred to as lingual tonsils. The anterior and posterior regions are separated by a shallow V-shaped groove known as the sulcus terminalis. The ventral surface of the tongue is lined by thin, nonkeratinized stratified squamous epithelium supported by a loose, highly vascular lamina propria.

Lingual Papillae of the Body of the Tongue

Filiform papillae

The filiform papillae are the most numerous type on the dorsum of the tongue. They are 1 to 3mm long and number in the thousands. They represent heavily keratinized, cone-shaped projections of overlapping sheets of superficial squamous cells extending above the surface. They give the tongue a rough-surface texture (Fig. 9-4-1). This type of papilla does not contain taste buds.

Fungiform papillae

The fungiform papillae are the second most numerous papillae. There are about 150 to 200 of these mushroom-shaped papillae randomly scattered on the dorsum of the tongue. They are about 2mm in diameter. They have a smooth surface of thinly keratinized stratified squamous epithelium (Figs. 9-4-1, 2; Fig. 9-5-1). The vascular connective tissue papillae gives them a red or pink color. They may contain several taste buds (Fig. 9-5-1).

Circumvallate papillae

The circumvallate papillae are found just anterior to and parallel with the sulcus terminalis (Fig. 9-1-1). The 10-12 papillae are about 1.5 to 3.0mm in diameter. The oral surface is covered by thinly keratinized stratified squamous epithelium. Their broad flat surface is surrounded by a circular trough or furrow (annular vallecula) lined by nonkeratinized stratified squamous epithelium (Fig. 9-5-2, Figs. 9-6-1, 2; Fig. 9-7-1). The epithelial surface of the papillae facing the trough is nonkeratinized epithelium with numerous taste buds.

Foliate papilla

The foliate papillae are found on the posterior lateral margin of the tongue. These papillae are rudimentary in humans, but there may be 2 to 16 in number (Fig. 9-7-2). These papillae are well-developed in the rabbit (Fig. 9-8-1). Here they are seen as vertical bulges on the mucous membrane with intervening grooves. The grooves are lined by nonkeratinized stratified squamous epithelium and contain numerous taste buds (Figs. 9-8-1, 2).

Taste Buds

The taste buds are associated with all four types of lingual papilla in fetuses older than 7 months and in the newborn infant. As the infant grows, the number of taste buds decrease in number, eventually disappearing in the filiform papilla. Each fungiform papilla may contain 3 to 4 taste buds (Fig. 9-5-1). Few, if any, taste buds are found in the foliate papillae of humans (Fig. 9-7-2). The circumvallate papillae contain numerous taste buds (Fig. 9-7-1). Taste buds may also be found in the palate, pharynx, larynx, esophagus, and epiglottis.

The taste buds are intra-epithelial chemoreceptors or organs of taste. They are barrel-shaped expansions that extend through the thickness of the epithelium to the surface (Fig. 9-9-1). At the surface there is a small opening or taste pore into the taste bud. The taste buds consist of neuroepithelial or taste cells (dark cells or Type I), sustentacular cells (light cell or Type II) and basal cells (Type VI) (Fig. 9-9-2). By electron microscopy, an intermediate light cell has been found and is designated as Type III cells. The taste cells have many long microvilli or taste hairs that extend toward the taste pore (Fig. 9-9-2). These three types of cells may represent different functional stages of the same cell. The basal cell (Type IV) may represent a germinal cell for the other cell types. Chemical synapses have been associated with only Type III cells.

The sensory innervation of the tongue is based on the contributions of the various pharyngeal or branchial arches. The body of the tongue is innervated by the lingual branch of the mandibular division of the trigeminal nerve (cranial nerve V). Taste reception from the fungiform papillae of the anterior two-thirds of the tongue are carried by the chorda tympani of the facial nerve (cranial nerve VII). The posterior one-third of the tongue, the circumvallate and the foliate papilla receive innervation from the glossopharyngeal nerve (cranial nerve IX).

Lingual salivary glands

All three types of salivary glands are represented in the tongue. The glands of von Ebner are pure serous glands that function to wash out the troughs of the circumvallate papillae and the interpapillary grooves of the foliate papillae (Fig. 9-8-1, Figs. 9-10-1, 2). Alveoli of pure serous cells will extend between the fascicles of the skeletal muscle of the tongue. The anterior lingual glands are mixed seromucous gland. The posterior lingual glands are pure mucous.

Mucous alveoli of this gland are also found between the muscle fascicles. Some glands on the root of the tongue may produce glycoproteins and may be designated as seromucous glands. Except for the glands of von Ebner, the ducts of the other glands open directly on the surface of the tongue.

Lingual tonsils

Posterior to the sulcus terminalis, the surface of the tongue is covered by numerous oval to round prominences called lingual follicles that comprise the lingual tonsil (Fig. 9-1-1). Many follicles have a small pit at the center known as the lingual crypt (Fig. 9-12-1). These elevations are due to the presence of lymphatic nodules in the lamina propria. Most of the lymphatic nodules have germinal centers (Figs. 9-11-1, 2; Fig. 9-12-1). Lymphocytes may migrate through the stratified squamous epithelium entering the oral cavity or enter the lymphatic vessels around the follicles. There are numerous blood vessels within the lamina propria (Fig. 9-12-2). Secretions from the minor submucosal mucous glands empty into the crypts.

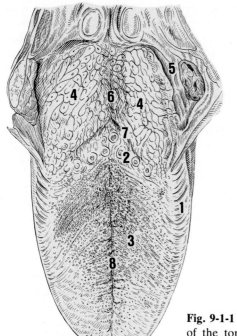

Fig. 9-1-1 Diagram of a surface view of the tongue.

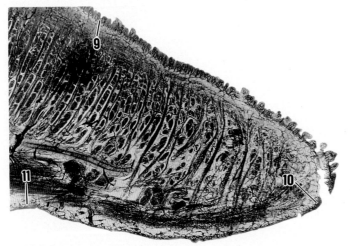

Fig. 9-1-2 Sagittal section of the tongue. India ink injected. X5

1. Foliate papillae
2. Circumvallate papillae
3. Filiform papillae and fungiform papillae
4. Lingual tonsils
5. Palatine tonsil

6. Foramen cecum
7. Sulcus terminalis
8. Median sulcus of the tongue
9↔10. Dorsum of the tongue
10↔11. Inferior surface of the tongue

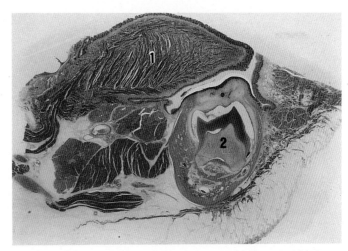

Fig. 9-2-1 Sagittal section of the tongue of a 1.5-year-old infant. H-E stain X2

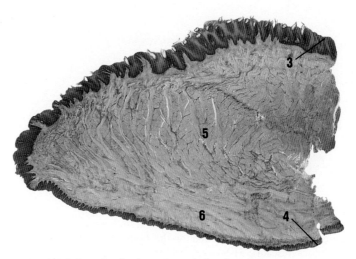

Fig. 9-2-2 Longitudinal section of the tip of the tongue (Macaca fuscata). H-E stain X15

1. Tongue
2. Mandibular molar tooth
3. Dorsum of the tongue
4. Inferior surface of the tongue
5. Transverse muscle of the tongue
6. Inferior longitudinal muscle of the tongue

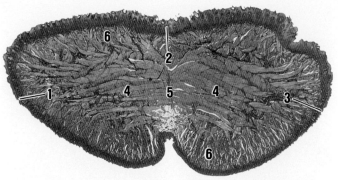

Fig. 9-3-1 Transverse section of the tip of the tongue (Macaca fuscata). H-E stain X15

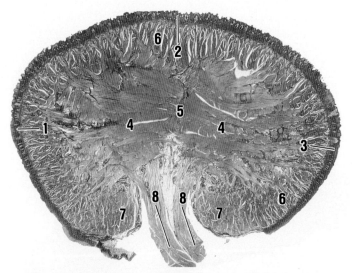

Fig. 9-3-2 Transverse section of the body of the tongue (Macaca fuscata). H-E stain X15

1↔2↔3. Dorsum of the tongue
  1↔3. Inferior surface of the tongue
    4. Transverse muscle of the tongue
    5. Medial septum of the tongue

6. Vertical muscle of the tongue
7. Inferior muscle of the tongue
8. Genioglossus muscle

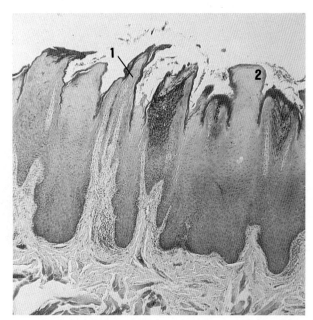

Fig. 9-4-1 Filiform papilla and fungiform papilla. H-E stain X80

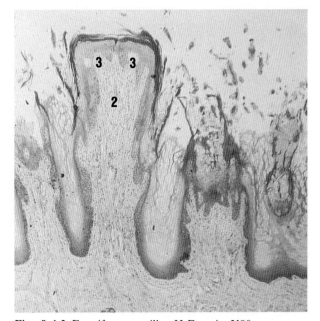

Fig. 9-4-2 Fungiform papilla. H-E stain X80

---

1. Filiform papilla

2. Fungiform papilla

3. Secondary connective tissue papilla

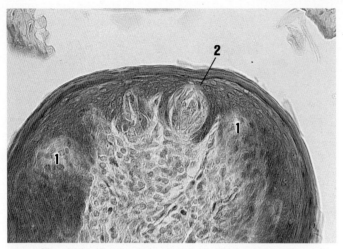

Fig. 9-5-1 Taste bud in a fungiform papilla. H-E stain X300

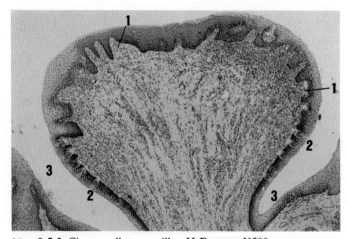

Fig. 9-5-2 Circumvallate papilla. H-E stain X500

1. Secondary connective tissue papilla
2. Taste bud
3. Trough or furrow (annular vallecula)

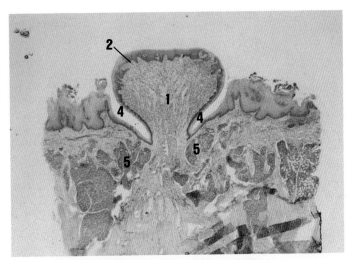

Fig. 9-6-1 Circumvallate papilla. H-E stain X20

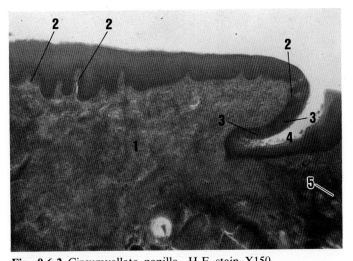

Fig. 9-6-2 Circumvallate papilla. H-E stain X150

1. Circumvallate papilla
2. Secondary connective tissue papilla
3. Taste bud
4. Trough
5. Glands of von Ebner

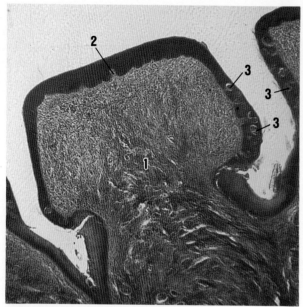

Fig. 9-7-1 Circumvallate papilla (Macaca fuscata). H-E stain X80

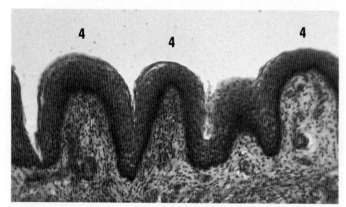

Fig. 9-7-2 Foliate papilla. H-E stain X100

---

1. Circumvallate papilla
2. Secondary connective tissue papilla
3. Taste bud
4. Foliate papilla

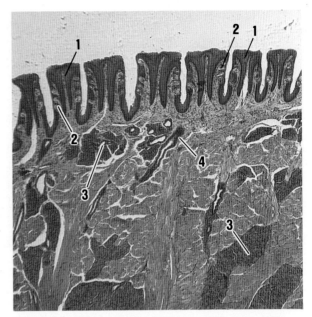

Fig. 9-8-1 Foliate papilla (Rabbit). H-E stain X40.

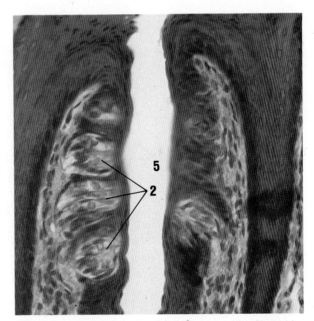

Fig. 9-8-2 Taste buds in the foliate papilla (Rabbit). H-E stain X800

1. Foliate papilla	4. Excretory duct of the gland of von Ebner
2. Taste bud	
3. Glands of von Ebner	5. Interpapillary groove

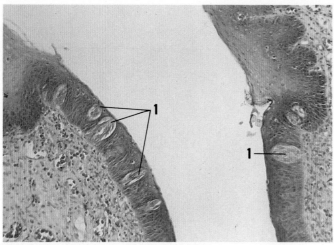

Fig. 9-9-1 Taste buds. H-E stain X800

It has been said that the taste cells (Type I) are long and slender with a dark elongated nucleus, while the sustentacular cells (Type II) are lighter with a pale rounded nucleus. An intermediate form of the light cells (Type III) is also found. Taste hairs or microvilli are seen in all three types. Synaptic vesicles are seen only in Type III cells. The basal cells (Type IV) are small germinal cells next to the connective tissue.

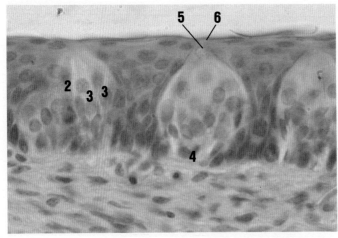

Fig. 9-9-2 Taste buds. H-E stain X1,200

1. Taste bud
2. Taste cell
3. Sustentacular cell
4. Basal cell
5. Taste canal
6. Taste pore

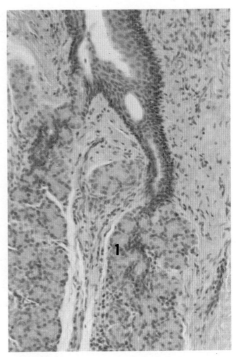

Fig. 9-10-1 Glands of von Ebner. H-E stain X200

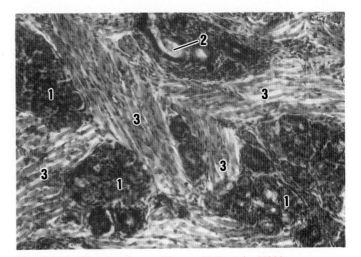

Fig. 9-10-2 Glands of von Ebner. H-E stain X200

1. Glands of von Ebner
2. Excretory duct of the glands of von Ebner

3. Muscles of the tongue

The lingual tonsils are comprised of numerous lymphatic nodules.

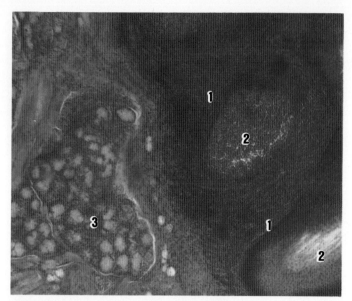

Fig. 9-11-1 Lymphatic nodule in the lingual tonsil. H-E stain X90

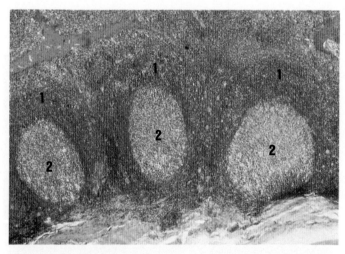

Fig. 9-11-2 Lymphatic nodules in the lingual tonsil. H-E stain X350

1. Lingual lymphatic follicle
2. Germinal center

3. Mucous glands in the root of the tongue

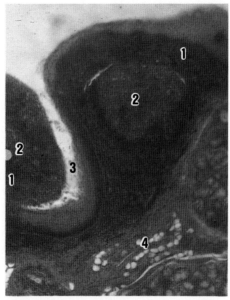

Fig. 9-12-1 Lymphatic nodule in lingual tonsil. H-E stain X70

1. Lymphatic nodule 2. Germinal center 3. Crypt of tonsil 4. Mucous glands in the root of the tongue

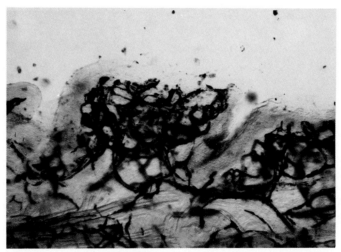

Fig. 9-12-2 Lingual papilla vascular injected with India ink. X200

10
Palate and Pharynx

PALATE AND PHARYNX

Palate

The palate is formed by the union of the two lateral palatine processes, the primary palate and the nasal septum. The development of bone within these structures separates the hard and soft palates.

Hard palate

The thick masticatory oral mucosa of the hard palate is covered by both keratinized and parakeratinized stratified squamous epithelium. It is supported by a lamina propria consisting of dense collagenous fiber bundles that tightly bind the mucosa to the bone of the palate. In the submucosal regions, these fiber bundles form thick partitions. There are three distinct mucosal regions of the hard palate. First, the mucosa of the anterior one-third is cast into elevated transverse folds or palatal rugae. The rugae are supported laterally by submucosal cushions of adipose tissue, thus forming a fatty anterior lateral zone. Second, in the posterior lateral two-thirds of the palate, the submucosa is filled with palatal salivary glands. This forms a glandular posterior lateral zone (Figs. 10-1-1, 2). Third, in the midline, the very thin, tough mucosa of the medial palatal raphe is bound directly to the bone in the form of a mucoperiosteum. This narrow region and the gingival portion of the hard palate lack a submucosa, glands and adipose tissue (Figs. 10-1-1, 2).

The palatal glands are minor mucous glands with short ducts that empty onto the epithelium of the hard palate (Fig. 10-2-2). These glands extend posteriorly into the submucosa beneath the oral mucous membrane of the soft palate.

In the midline, immediately posterior to the maxillary central incisors is the incisive papilla. This small projection of tissue is composed of dense connective tissue that may contain small islands of cartilage. It overlies the oral opening of the incisive canal (Fig. 10-2-1). The canal contains the nasopalatine nerve and blood vessels, and remnants of the nasopalatine ducts. The nasopalatine ducts are vestigial in humans, being functional in lower mammals as part of Jacobson's organ of olfaction.

Soft palate

The lack of a core of bone in the soft palate makes this tissue soft and flexible. The posterior free surface, in the midline, is extended to form the uvula. The lining oral mucosa of the soft palate is composed of nonkeratinized stratified squamous epithelium and supported by a loose fibro-elastic connective tissue. A dense band of elastic fibers, in the form of an elastic lamina, divides the lamina propria from the glandular submucosa. This lamina is pierced by nerves, blood vessels and the small excretory ducts of minor salivary glands. The submucosa contains numerous mucous-secreting glands. Glandular tissue may extend between the fascicles of skeletal muscle that forms the central region of the soft palate (Figs. 10-3-1, 2; Fig. 10-4-1). The soft palate serves as the attachment for several skeletal muscles arising from the palate and pharynx.

The superior surface of the soft palate is covered by respiratory mucosa. The ciliated pseudostratified epithelium with goblet cells is supported by a thin lamina propria. Small seromucous glands are located within a thin submucosa and empty onto the surface of the nasal mucosa (Fig. 10-4-2).

Pharynx

The pharynx is a fibromuscular tube extending between the nasal chambers and the oral cavity above and the larynx below. Thus, it can be divided into three regions: nasopharynx, oropharynx, and laryngopharynx. The nasopharynx receives the openings of both the auditory tube and the posterior nasal chambers. The wall of the pharynx is composed of a mucosa, a muscle layer or muscularis and an outer coat of connective tissue or an adventitia.

The greater part of the pharynx is lined by nonkeratinized stratified squamous epithelium. Parts of the nasopharynx are lined by ciliated pseudostratified columnar epithelium containing goblet cells.

The pharyngeal glands are both mucous and seromucous in type. The seromucous glands are mainly found in the regions covered by ciliated epithelium of the nasopharynx, while the mucous glands are found underneath the epithelium in the other regions of the pharynx (Fig. 10-4-3).

The lamina propria of the pharynx contain masses of lymphatic tissue or tonsils. These are located between the palatoglossal and palatopharyngeal arches (palatine tonsils), the distal wall of the nasopharynx (pharyngeal tonsil) and around the openings of the auditory canals (tubal or Gerlach's tonsil). The lamina propria of the pharynx also contains a thick elastic lamina similar to that seen in the soft palate. This layer separates the lamina propria from the layer of constrictor muscles and other pharyngeal muscles. It may extend between the fascicles of muscle. In the esophagus, the elastic lamina is replaced by the muscularis mucosa. Outside of the muscle layer of the pharyngeal wall, dense connective tissue in the form of an adventitia blends with the connective tissue of adjacent structures.

Tonsils

The palatine tonsils are bilateral ovoid lymphatic structures situated in the tonsillar sinus between the palatoglossal and the palatopharyngeal arches. Each tonsil is about one inch in length by one-half inch in width. They are orientated parallel with the pharyngeal fauces. The oral surface of the tonsil is deeply infolded in the form of branching crypts. Nonkeratinized stratified squamous epithelium lines the surface of the tonsil and extends into the crypts. Deep within the crypts the epithelium may be com-

pletely eroded by lymphatic cells. The lamina propria is filled with numerous lymphatic nodules, most of which display both a cortical region and a germinal center (Fig. 10-5). Beneath the lymphatic tissue, the fibrous connective tissue of the lamina propria forms an loose capsule. Seromucous glands may be found in the submucosa. Most of the excretory ducts open onto the surface of the tonsil.

The pharyngeal tonsil or adenoids are similar in structure to the palatine tonsils with the following exceptions: the surface is infolded in the form of longitudinal folds and the surface is lined by ciliated epithelium. A thin capsule is present as well as seromucous glands.

The palatine, pharyngeal and lingual tonsils form an incomplete ring of lymphatic tissue around the entrance to the pharynx. This arrangement is sometimes referred to as Waldeyer's ring.

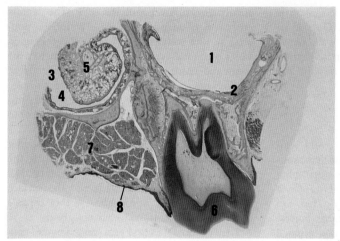

Fig. 10-1-1 Frontal section of the hard palate. H-E stain X2

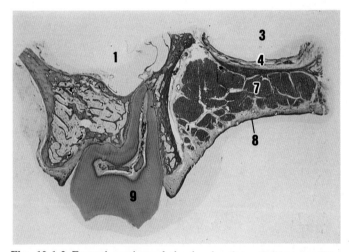

Fig. 10-1-2 Frontal section of the hard palate. H-E stain X2

1. Maxillary sinus
2. Mucosa of maxillary sinus
3. Nasal cavity
4. Nasal mucous membrane
5. Inferior nasal concha
6. Maxillary second molar
7. Palatine mucous glands
8. Palatal mucous membrane
9. Maxillary first molar

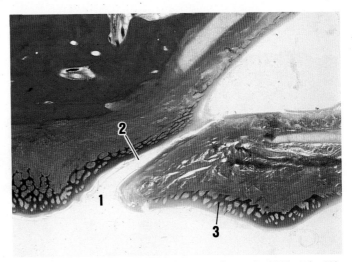

Fig. 10-2-1 Nasopalatine duct (Macaca fuscata). H-E stain X8

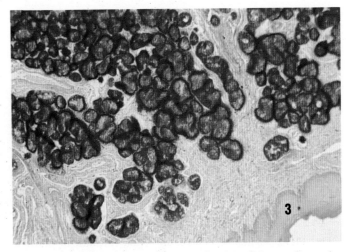

Fig. 10-2-2 Mucous glands in the hard palate (Macaca fuscata). PAS stain X170

1. Oral opening of the nasopalatine duct
2. Nasopalatine duct
3. Epithelium of the palatal mucous membrane

207

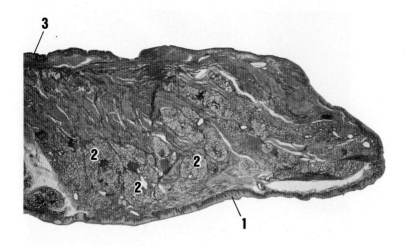

Fig. 10-3-1 Soft palate (Macaca fuscata). H-E stain X4

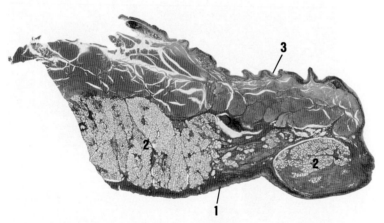

Fig. 10-3-2 Sagittal section of the uvula (Macaca fuscata). H-E stain X4

1. Stratified squamous epithelium of the palatal mucous membrane
2. Mucous glands of the palate
3. Ciliated pseudostratified columnar epithelium of the nasal mucosa

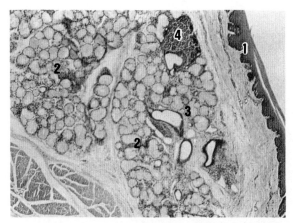

Fig. 10-4-1 Glands in the soft palate (Macaca fuscata). H-E stain X40

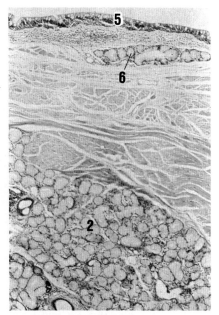

Fig. 10-4-2 Nasal mucous membrane in the soft palate (Macaca fuscata). H-E stain X40

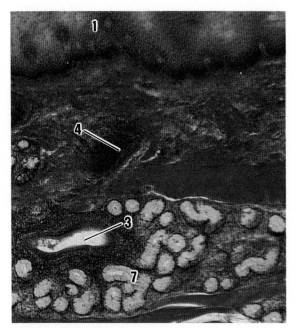

Fig. 10-4-3 Pharyngeal mucous membrane (Macaca fuscata). H-E stain X40

1. Nonkeratinized stratified squamous epithelium
2. Mucous glands of the palate
3. Excretory duct
4. Lymph nodule

5. Ciliated pseudostratified columnar epithelium of the nasal mucosa
6. Seromucous glands in the nasal mucosa
7. Seromucous glands in the pharyngeal mucosa

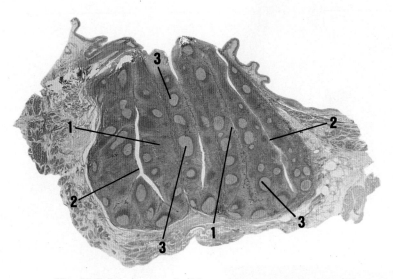

Fig. 10-5 Palatine tonsil (Macaca fuscata). H-E stain X8

1. Lymph follicles or nodules
2. Tonsillar crypts

3. Germinal center

11
Maxillary Sinuses

MAXILLARY SINUS

The maxillary sinus is a pneumatic space within the maxilla that communicates with the nasal cavity. It is formed as an outgrowth of the nasal epithelium from the lateral wall of the middle meatus. The mucous membrane of the maxillary sinus is a continuation of the nasal mucosa. It is, however, somewhat thinner than that of the nasal cavity. The ciliated pseudostratified columnar epithelium is reduced in height with fewer goblet cells. The lamina propria is thinner with fewer and smaller seromucous glands in comparison with the nasal mucosa (Fig. 11-3).

The inferior border or floor of the maxillary sinus is in close association with the root apices of the maxillary posterior teeth. The sinus is most commonly associated with the roots of the maxillary first molars (Figs. 11-1-1, 2). The apical tips of the roots are usually separated from the sinus by a thin plate of bone, however, soft tissue communication may also exist (Fig. 11-2-1).

The superior alveolar neurovascular bundle passes along the floor of the sinus within the submucosal tissue. Pressure or inflammation within the maxillary sinus may produce pain or even paresthesia. Due to the close proximity of the roots of the teeth and the sinus, any inflammation of the sinus may spread to the teeth and the expansion of an apical abscess may produce a maxillary sinusitis (Fig. 11-2-2).

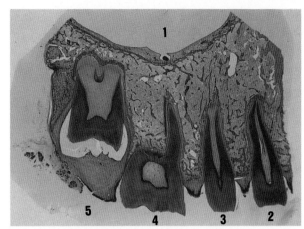

Fig. 11-1-1 Sagittal sections showing the positional relation of the maxillary sinus to the roots of the maxillary posterior teeth. H-E stain X3

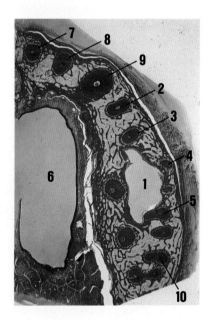

Fig. 11-1-2 Horizontal section showing the positional relation of the maxillary sinus to the roots of the maxillary teeth. H-E stain X3

1. Maxillary sinus
2. Maxillary first premolar
3. Maxillary second premolar
4. Maxillary first molar
5. Maxillary second molar

6. Nasal cavity
7. Maxillary central incisor
8. Maxillary lateral incisor
9. Maxillary canine
10. Maxillary third molar

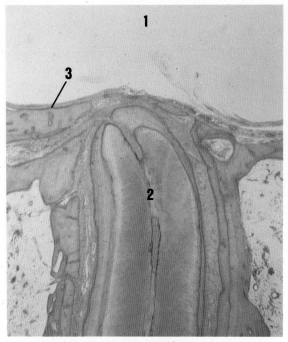

Fig. 11-2-1 Relation of the maxillary sinus to the root apex of a maxillary molar. H-E stain X20

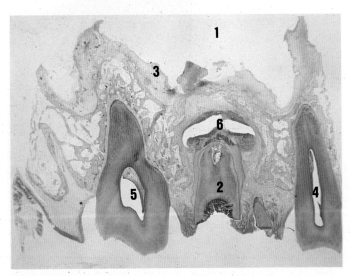

Fig. 11-2-2 Sagittal sections of a maxillary sinusitis of odontogenic origin. H-E stain X3

1. Maxillary sinus
2. Lingual root of the maxillary first molar
3. Mucosa of the floor of the maxillary sinus
4. Maxillary second premolar
5. Maxillary second molar
6. Apical abscess

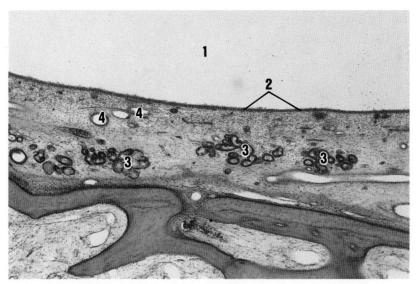

Fig. 11-3 Mucous membrane of the maxillary sinus. H-E stain X80

1. Maxillary sinus
2. Ciliated pseudostratified columnar epithelium of the maxillary sinus
3. Seromucous glands
4. Excretory ducts of a seromucous gland

12

Maxillary and Mandibular Bones

MAXILLA AND MANDIBLE

Mandible

The primordium of the mandible appears on the lateral side of Meckel's cartilage during the middle of the 6th week of embryonic development. The bone of the body of the mandible forms by intramembranous ossification. Mineralization of the primitive bone begins during the 7th week (Figs. 12-1-1, 2). The primitive mandible is termed the os dentale. Bone forms anterior to the branch of the incisive and mental nerves and spreads both anteriorly toward the midline and posteriorly toward the branch of the inferior alveolar and lingual nerves. It forms along the lateral aspect of Meckel's cartilage forming a trough consisting of medial and lateral plates that unite beneath the incisal nerve (Fig. 1-E). The trough is soon formed into a canal as bone forms over the nerve joining the medial and lateral plates. The ramus of the mandible begins to form during the 7th week of development.

The coronoid and condylar processes are formed by endochondral ossification. The coronoid growth cartilage appears at about 14 weeks and disappears by the 20th week. The coronoid process is mineralized by the seventh month and fuses with the body of the mandible. The condylar cartilage is seen at about 3 months and will persist until the end of the second decade. It will form as a component of the temporomandibular joint. Thus the mandible is formed by both intramembranous and endochondral ossification, whereas the maxilla is formed only by intramembranous ossification.

Maxilla

At the end of the 6th week the incisive bone of the globular process appears (Fig. 1-7-2). The primitive maxilla appears by the end of the 7th week soon after the appearance of the mandible (Fig. 1-6-2, Fig. 12-1-2). Mineralization begins a few days later (Fig. 1-8-1, Fig. 12-3-1). The incisive bone is still separated from the maxillary bone until the end of the 7th week (Fig. 1-7-2, Fig. 12-3-1). They will later fuse with each other (Fig. 12-A). The incisive bone contains the four incisor tooth buds while the maxilla contains the cuspid and the other posterior tooth buds. The bone of the palate appears within the fused lateral palatine processes at the beginning of the 7th week of development (Fig 12-A, Fig. 12-1-1, Fig. 12-3-1). Fusion with the maxillary bone occurs during the 14th week (Fig. 12-3-2). The palatine bone does not contain teeth (Figs. 12-5-1, 2; Fig. 12-6-1).

Meckel's Cartilage

The cartilage of the first branchial arch, Meckel's cartilage, appears during the 6th week as a solid bar of cartilage extending from the region of the ear to the midline of the fused mandibular processes. These two bars do not meet at the midline but are separated from each other by mesenchyme. Meckel's cartilage resides lingual to the developing mandible (Fig. 1-E, Fig. 12-4-2). With the development of the mandible, the cartilage degenerates beginning near the midline and continues in a posterior direction (Fig. 1-13- 2). The most posterior portion, however, remains to form two ossicles of the ear, the malleus and the incus. The perichondrium remains as the sphenomandibular ligament. Meckel's cartilage does not participate in the formation of the mandible.

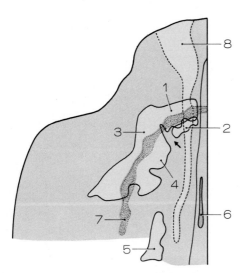

Fig. 12-A Horizontally-sectioned graphic reconstruction diagram of the maxilla of a 9-week human fetus (40mm CR length).

1. Incisive alveolar ridge **2.** Premaxilla **3.** Maxilla **4.** Maxillary palate **5.** Palatine bone **6.** Vomer bone **7.** Dental lamina **8.** Nasal cavity **9.** Globulomaxillary suture

The ossifying mandibular primordium is called the os dentale. At 43 days of development of the mandible is advanced.

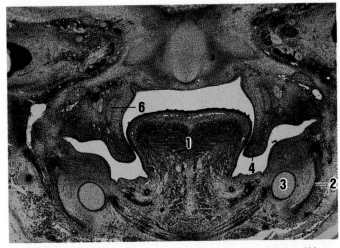

Fig. 12-1-1 Frontal section of a 43-day human embryo (20mm CR length). Development of the mandibular and palatine bones. Masson stain X4

In the region of the molar teeth, Meckel's cartilage resides on the lingual side of the developing mandible.

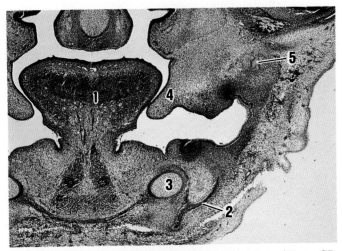

Fig. 12-1-2 Frontal section of a 45-day human embryo (26mm CR length). Development of the primitive mandible and Meckel's cartilage. Masson stain X4

1. Tongue
2. Primordium of the mandibular bone (Os dentale)
3. Meckel's cartilage
4. Lateral palatine process
5. Primordium of the maxillary bone
6. Primordium of the palatine bone

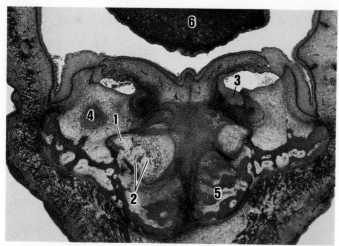

Meckel's cartilage is in the process of degeneration. Blood vessels are seen invading the cartilage matrix. In this incisor region, the mandible appears in close relation to Meckel's cartilage.

Fig. 12-2-1 Frontal section of a 11-week human fetus (71mm CR length). Meckel's cartilage and mandible. Azan stain X30

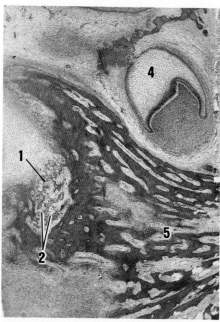

Fig. 12-2-2 Frontal section of a 13-week human fetus. Meckel's cartilage and mandible. H-E stain X37

1. Degenerating Meckel's cartilage
2. Blood vessels
3. Primary mandibular central incisor tooth germ
4. Primary mandibular lateral incisor tooth germ
5. Mandible
6. Tongue

The forming maxilla and palatine bones develop separately until the end of the 6th week of development. In some regions, they overlap each other. During the 15th week, they fuse with each other.

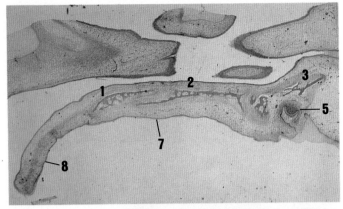

Fig. 12-3-1 Parasagittal section of a 11-week human fetus (73mm CR length). Masson stain X10.5

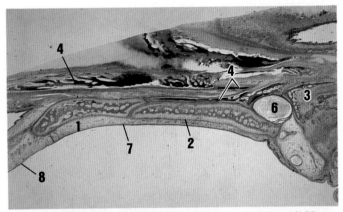

Fig. 12-3-2 Parasagittal section of a 18-week human fetus (155mm CR length). Masson stain X10

1. Palatine bone
2. Maxillary bone
3. Incisive bone
4. Vomer bone
5. Primary maxillary incisor tooth germ
6. Nasopalatine duct
7. Hard palate
8. Soft palate

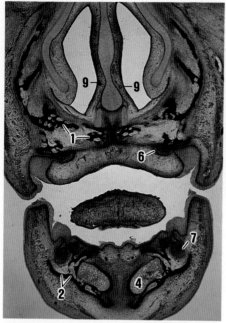

Fig. 12-4-1 Frontal section of a 9-week human fetus (45mm CR length). Azan stain X13

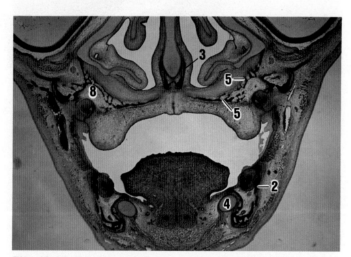

Fig. 12-4-2 Frontal section of a 9-week human fetus (45mm CR length). Azan stain X13

1. Incisive bone
2. Mandibular bone
3. Vomer bone
4. Meckel's cartilage
5. Maxillary bone

6. Primary maxillary lateral incisor tooth germ
7. Primary mandibular canine tooth germ
8. Primary maxillary first molar tooth germ
9. Jacobson's organ

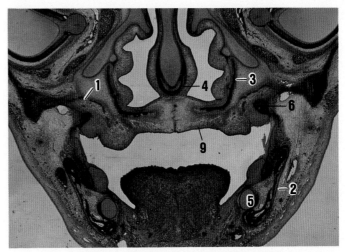

Fig. 12-5-1 Frontal section of a 9-week human fetus (45mm CR length). Azan stain X13

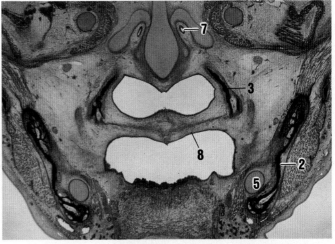

Fig. 12-5-2 Frontal section of a 9-week human fetus (45mm CR length). Azan stain X13

1. Maxillary bone
2. Mandibular bone
3. Palatine bone
4. Vomer bone
5. Meckel's cartilage
6. Primary maxillary second molar tooth germ
7. Sphenoidal sinus
8. Soft palate
9. Hard palate

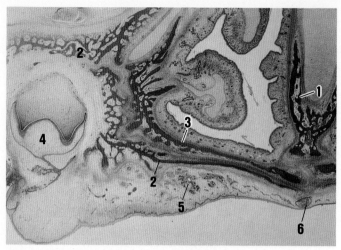

Fig. 12-6-1 Frontal section of a 16-week human fetus. H-E stain X14

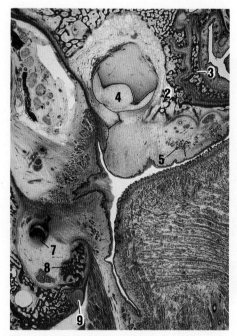

Fig. 12-6-2 Frontal section of a 16-week human fetus. H-E stain X14

1. Vomer bone
2. Maxillary bone
3. Palatine bone
4. Primary maxillary second molar tooth germ
5. Palatine glands
6. Epithelial rests within fused margins of palatine processes
7. Secondary mandibular first molar tooth germ
8. Mandibular bone
9. Meckel's cartilage

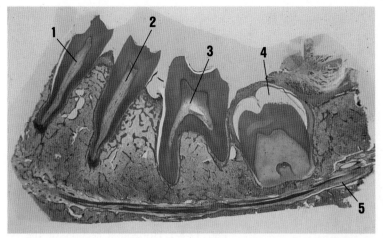

Fig. 12-7-1 Sagittal section of the mandible of a 12 year old child. H-E stain X3

1. Mandibular first premolar 2. Mandibular second premolar 3. Mandibular first molar 4. Mandibular second molar 5. Mandibular canal

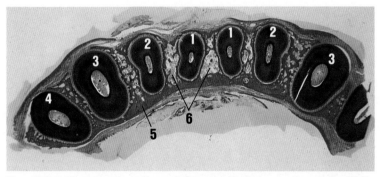

Fig. 12-7-2 Horizontal section of the mandibular anterior teeth. H-E stain X3

1. Root of mandibular central incisor 2. Root of mandibular lateral incisor 3. Root of mandibular canine 4. Root of mandibular first premolar 5. Lingual cortical plate of the mandible 6. Spongy bone of the interalveolar septum

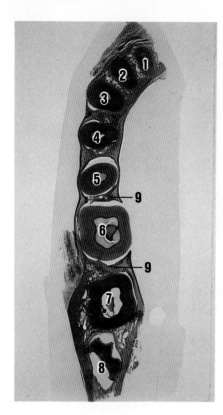

Fig. 12-8-1 Horizontal section of the mandible. H-E stain X2

1. Root of mandibular central incisor 2. Root of mandibular lateral incisor 3. Root of mandibular canine 4. Root of mandibular first premolar 5. Root of mandibular second premolar 6. Root of mandibular first molar 7. Root of mandibular second molar 8. Mandibular third molar tooth germ 9. Interalveolar septum

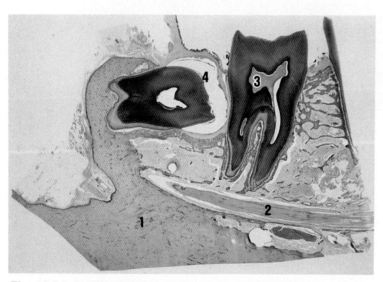

Fig. 12-8-2 Sagittal section of an horizontally-positioned mandibular third molar. H-E stain X2

1. Mandible 2. Inferior alveolar nerve 3. Mandibular second molar 4. Mandibular third molar

13

Temporomandibular Joint

TEMPOROMANDIBULAR JOINT

The temporomandibular joint is a bilateral diarthrosis between the mandibular condyles and the articular tubercle (anteriorly) and the mandibular or glenoid fossa (posteriorly) of the temporal bone. It begins to form during the 10th week and does not reach mature dimensions until the start of the second decade. Within the joint between the condylar head and the temporal bone is an articular disc (Fig. 13-1-1). Between the articulating surface of the temporal bone and the superior surface of the articular disc is the temporodiscal or superior synovial cavity. Between the inferior surface of the articular disc and the superior surface of the articulating surface of the mandibular condyle is the condylodiscal or inferior synovial cavity (Figs. 13-1-1, 2).

The articular disc is biconcave in shape and composed of dense collagenous connective tissue. The intermediate region of the biconcave disc is the thinnest part. This region is also avascular and lacks nerve fibers. The anterior region is continuous with the articular capsule and the fascia and tendon of the superior belly of the lateral pterygoid muscle. The posterior region is continuous with the loose fibro-elastic connective tissue known as the retroarticular cushion or bilaminar zone (Fig. 13-1-1). In this zone, the upper layer is attached to the temporal bone by a dense band of fibro-elastic connective tissue. The fibrous lower layer is attached to the posterior neck of the condyle. Between these two layers is adipose connective tissue containing blood vessels and nerves. With advancing age, cartilage cells or small islands of hyaline cartilage may be found within the disc.

The capsule of the joint extends anteriorly from the neck of the condyle to the articular tubercle of the temporal bone. Laterally, the capsule is thickened to form the temporomandibular ligament. The joint cavity is lined by a synovial membrane with synovial villi on nonarticulating surfaces. Some synovial villi contain unmyelinated nerve fibers.

The head of the mandibular condyle is composed of typical spongy or cancellous bone covered by a thin layer of compact bone (Figs. 13-2-1, 2). The articulating surface of the condyle is covered by a thick, dense fibrous perichondrium (Fig. 13-2-2, Fig. 13-4). Between the compact bone and the articular layer of connective tissue is a layer of hyaline cartilage (Fig. 13-2-2, Figs. 13-3-1, 2). In the young, the bone marrow is hemopoietic. With advancing age, the bone marrow is filled with adipose tissue.

The roof of the mandibular fossa is a thin plate of compact bone (Fig. 13-2-1). The articular tubercle is composed of spongy bone covered by a thin layer of compact bone. Both articulating areas are covered by dense fibrous tissue (Fig. 13-4). The fibrous layer covering the articulating surface of the fossa is thin but rapidly thickens on the posterior slope of the articular tubercle. The fibrous lining is bilayered: an inner layer with the fiber orientation perpendicular to the bone surface, and an outer layer where the fibers are parallel to the surface. With advancing age, cartilage cells may be found in this fibrous layer.

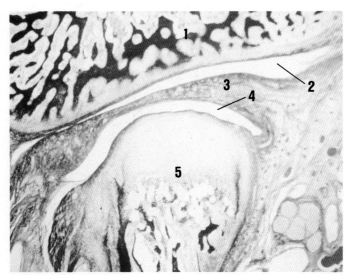

Fig. 13-1-1 Formation of the temporomandibular joint in a 5-month human fetus. H-E stain X4

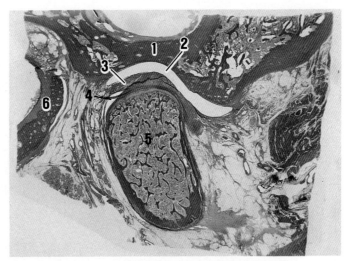

Fig. 13-1-2 Temporomandibular joint. H-E stain X4

1. Mandibular or glenoid fossa of the temporal bone
2. Superior (temporodiscal) synovial cavity
3. Articular disc
4. Inferior (condylodiscal) synovial cavity
5. Condylar head of the mandible
6. Mastoid process

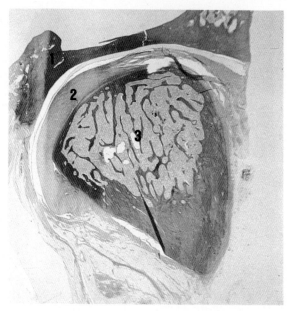

Fig. 13-2-1 Temporomandibular joint. H-E stain X5
1. Temporal bone 2. Articular disc 3. Condylar head of the mandible

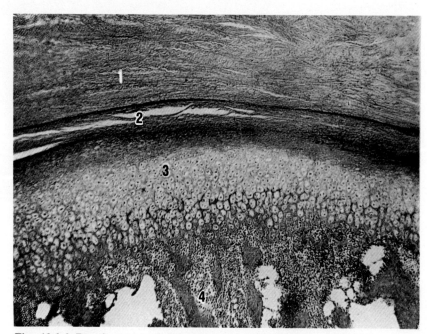

Fig. 13-2-2 Development of the temporomandibular joint. X44
1. Articular disc 2. Perichondrium 3. Hyaline cartilage 4. Hemopoietic bone marrow

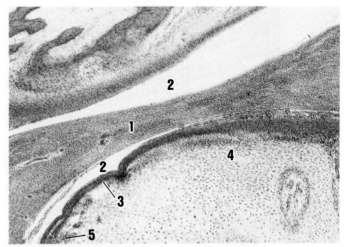

Fig. 13-3-1 Hyaline layer of the mandibular condyle. H-E stain X97

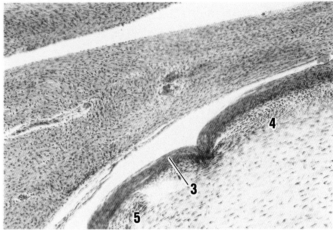

Fig. 13-3-2 Hyaline layer of the mandibular condyle. H-E stain X195

1. Articular disc
2. Synovial cavity
3. Fibrous covering
4. Hyaline cartilage
5. Calcified zone

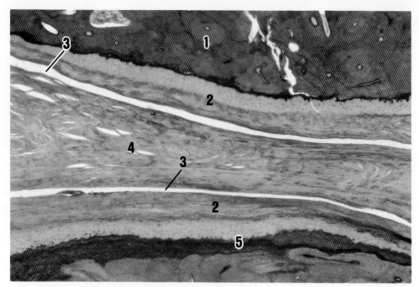

Fig. 13-4 Articular disc. H-E stain X195

1. Mandibular or glenoid fossa of temporal bone
2. Fibrous covering of temporal bone
3. Inferior synovial cavity
4. Articular disc
5. Head of mandibular condyle

14

Osteogenesis

OSTEOGENESIS

There are two methods of bone formation: endochondral ossification and intramembranous ossification. In endochondral ossification a growth plate of hyaline cartilage is first calcified then covered by bone (Figs. 14-1-1, 2). Parts of the mandible and the skull form by this method.

Intramembranous ossification involves the condensation of mesenchyme which leads to the differentiation of bone-forming cells, the osteoblasts. Bone is formed directly in the mesenchyme (Figs. 14-4-1, 2). The maxilla and the major portions of the sphenoid, temporal, occipital and mandible are formed by this method.

The embryonic periosteum around the bone is composed of two layers: a thick inner osteogenic or cambium and a thinner outer fibrous layer (Figs. 14-2-1, 2; Fig. 14-3-1). The cambial layer contains undifferentiated bone cells or osteoprogenitor cells and osteoblasts (Fig. 14-2-2, Fig. 14-3-2). Osteoblasts line the surface of the bone and produce osteoid, the unmineralized matrix, which later mineralizes. Osteocytes are osteoblasts that became embedded in bone. They reside within lacuna and maintain contact with the surface via long cytoplasmic processes that course within canaliculi (Fig. 14-5). The osteoclast, a multinucleated giant cell, functions in the resorption of bone (Fig. 14-3-2). The active osteoclast creates a depression on the surface of the bone called a Howship's lacuna. The outer fibrous layer of the embryonic periosteum is composed of undifferentiated mesenchymal cells and fibroblasts (Figs. 14-2-1, 2; Fig. 14-3-1).

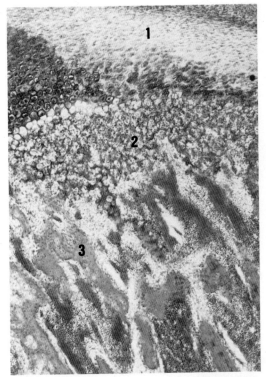

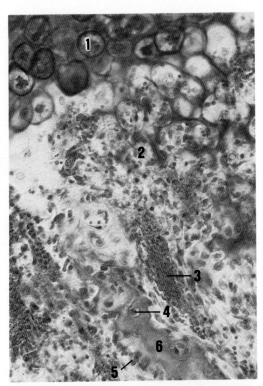

Fig. 14-1-1 Endochondral bone formation with hyaline cartilage. H-E stain X200

1. Perichondrium 2. Hyaline cartilage 3. Calcified bone

Fig. 14-1-2 Higher magnification of part of Fig. 14-1-1 showing replacement of calcified hyaline cartilage by bone. H-E stain X400

1. Hyaline cartilage 2. Resorbing cartilage 3. Blood vessel 4. Osteocyte 5. Osteoblast 6. Calcified bone

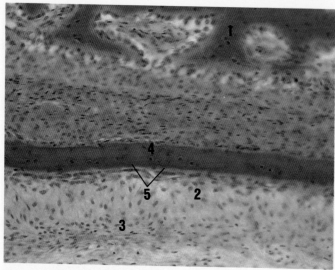

Fig. 14-2-1 Frontal section of a 12-week human fetus showing membranous bone. H-E stain X144

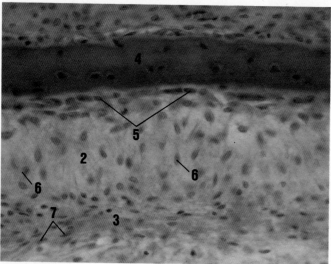

Fig. 14-2-2 Enlargement of part of Fig. 14-2-1 showing the embryonic periosteum. H-E stain X216

1. Palatine bone
2. Osteogenic (cambial) layer of periosteum
3. Fibrogenic (capsular) layer of periosteum
4. Maxillary bone
5. Osteoblast
6. Fibroblast
7. Fibrocyte

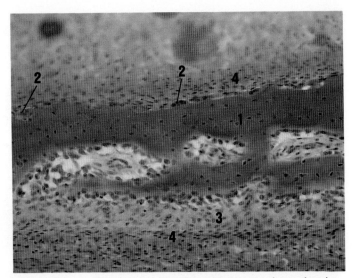

Fig. 14-3-1 Frontal section of a 12-week human fetus showing membranous bone formation. H-E stain X144

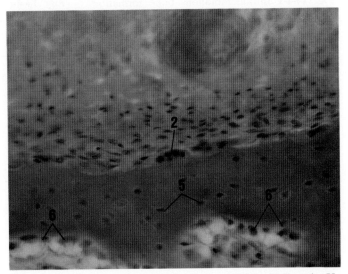

Fig. 14-3-2 Enlargement of part of Fig. 14-3-1. H-E stain X 216

1. Palatine bone
2. Osteoclast
3. Osteogenic (cambial) layer of the periosteum
4. Fibrogenic (capsular) layer of the periosteum
5. Osteocyte
6. Osteoblast

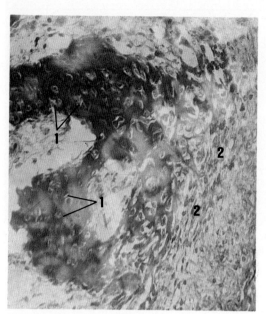

Fig. 14-4-1 Intramembranous bone formation. Azan stain X400

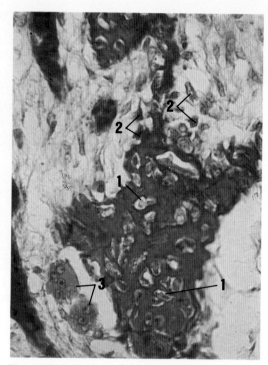

Fig. 14-4-2 Intramembranous bone formation. Azan stain X400

1. Osteocytes
2. Osteoblasts

3. Osteoclasts

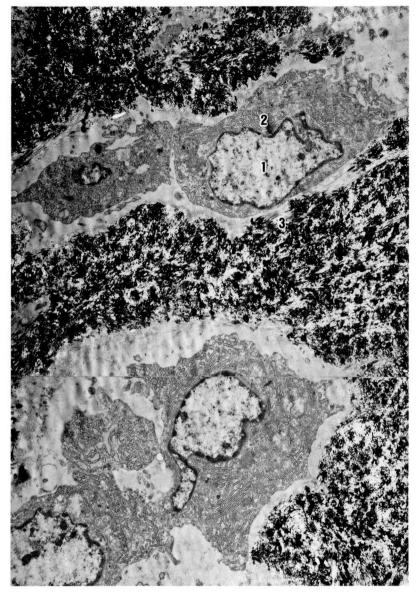

Fig. 14-5 Transmission electron micrograph of osteocytes in lacuna. X3,570

1. Nucleus
2. Golgi complex
3. Collagen fibers

INDEX*

*Bold face page numbers indicate a listing found in the text. Regular face page numbers indicate
listings found in the figure legends.

seromucous glands
    Minor **161**
        buccal 164, **180**, 184, 185
        labial 164, **180**, 181, 182
        lingual **189**
        nasal **204**, 209, **212**, 215
        pharyngeal **204**, **205**, 209
        retromolar **180**
    parotid **160**
    sublingual **161**
    submandibular **160**
seromucous salivary cell **160**, 178
    serous demilune 182, 185, 186
    serous glands of von Ebner **160**, **161**, **189**, 195, 197, 199
    Sharpey's fibers in
    bone 124, 126, **136**, **137**
    cementum 124, 126, 129, 130, **136**, 141
sinus
    maxillary 206, **212**, 213, 214, 215
    sphenoid 19, 223
soft palate 2, **204**, 208, 209, 221, 223
sphenoidal sinus 19, 223
sphenomandibular ligament **218**
stellate reticulum **6**, 22, 23, 24, 29, 32, 33, 36, 38
Stenson's duct (parotid gland) **160**, 162
stomodeum 2, 10, 11, 12, 13, 14
stratified squamous epithelium **136**, **180**, 184, **188**, **204**, **205**, 208, 209
stratum intermedium **6**, 29, 32, 33, 36, 36, 38
striae of Retzius **54**, 59, 65
striated duct **160**, **161**, 165, 166, 169, 170, 172, 174, 175
styloglossus muscle 163, **188**
sublingual papilla (caruncula sublingualis) **161**
sublingual salivary gland **161**, 175, 176, 177, 178

submandibular ganglion 163
submandibular salivary gland **160**, 169, 170, 171, 172, 173, 174
successional dental lamina 20, 23, 24
sulcular epithelium **136**, 154, 155
sulcus,
    gingival (see gingival sulcus)
    of tongue 190
sulcus terminalis **188**, 190
superior labial tubercle (ridge) **7**
sustentacular cell **188**, 198
sweat glands **180**
synovial cavity 231
    condylodiscal **228**, 229, 232
    temporodiscal **228**, 229
synovial membrane **228**

T

taste bud **188**, 194, 195, 196, 197, 198
taste (gustatory) canal 198
taste (gustatory) cells **188**, 198
taste hairs **188**
taste (gustatory) pore **188**, 198
temporal bone **228**, 229, 230, 232
temporomandibular joint **218**, **228**, 229, 230
temporomandibular ligament **228**
tertiary (reparative) dentin **73**, 94, 96, 97, 98, **106**, 126
third molar
    mandibular 225, 226
    maxillary 47, 49, 213
Tomes' granular layer **73**, 92, 93, 129
Tomes' dentinal process (fiber) 34, 35, **72**, **106**
tongue 11, 12, 13, 14, 18, 19, 21, 26, 28, **160**, **161**, 163, **188**, **189**, 190, 191, 192, 219, 220
tonofibril 158
tonsils
    lingual **189**, 190, 200, 201

palatine **205**, 210
    pharyngeal (adenoids) **204**, **205**, 223
tonsillar crypt
    lingual **189**, 201
    palatine **205**, 210
tooth bud (germ) 20, 25, 46
transparent dentin **73**, 98, 99, 100
transseptal fibers **136**, 140, 144
tufts, enamel **55**, 58, 66

U

undifferentiated mesenchymal cells (see mesenchyme) **106**, **234**
unmyelinated nerve fiber 119
uvula **204**, 208

V

vallate (circumvallate) papilla **188**, 190, 194, 195, 196
vermillion border of lip **180**, 181
vestibular lamina **6**, 15, 16
vestibule, labial/buccal **6**
vomer bone 16, 17
vomeronasal organ (Jacobson's) 20
von Ebner
    incremental lines of **72**, 85
    glands of **160**, **161**, **189**, 195, 197, 199

W

Waldeyer's (lymphatic) ring **205**
Weil, zone of **106**, 108, 110, 113
Wharton's duct (submandibular gland) **161**, 163
wisdom tooth 226

Z

zone of Weil **106**, 108, 110, 113
zymogen (secretory) granules **160**, 167, 168